Office Management of Colon and Rectal Disease

GUY L. KRATZER, M.D.
Chief, Colon and Rectal Surgery
Allentown and Sacred Heart Hospitals
Allentown, Pennsylvania
Clinical Professor of Surgery
Hershey Medical Center
Hershey, Pennsylvania

ROBERT J. DEMAREST
Director, Audio-Visual Services
College of Physicians and Surgeons
  of Columbia University
New York, New York

1985
W.B. SAUNDERS COMPANY
Philadelphia   London   Toronto   Mexico City   Rio de Janeiro   Sydney   Tokyo

W. B. Saunders Company: West Washington Square
Philadelphia, PA   19105

1 St. Anne's Road
Eastbourne, East Sussex BN21 3UN, England

1 Goldthorne Avenue
Toronto, Ontario M8Z 5T9, Canada

Apartado 26370—Cedro 512
Mexico 4, D.F., Mexico

Rua Coronel Cabrita, 8
Sao Cristovao Caixa Postal 21176
Rio de Janeiro, Brazil

9 Waltham Street
Artarmon, N.S.W. 2064, Australia

Ichibancho, Central Bldg., 22-1 Ichibancho
Chiyoda-Ku, Tokyo 102, Japan

Library of Congress Cataloging in Publication Data

Kratzer, Guy L.

Office management of colon and rectal disease.

1. Colon (Anatomy)—Surgery.   2. Rectum—Surgery.
   3. Colon (Anatomy)—Diseases—Treatment.   4. Rectum—
Diseases—Treatment.   I. Title. [DNLM: 1. Colonic diseases.   2. Rectal diseases.   3. Ambulatory surgery. WI
600 K89o]

RD541.K73 1985   617'.5547   84–1392

ISBN 0–7216–1189–3

Office Management of Colon and Rectal Disease   ISBN   0-7216-1189-3

Last digit is the print number: 9   8   7   6   5   4   3   2   1

Foreword

In this timely book, Dr. Kratzer has given us the benefit of a wealth of experience in the diagnosis and management of anorectal and colonic disease. He systematically approaches his topics, beginning with anatomy and ending, interestingly and informatively, with the role of diet. An entire detailed chapter is devoted to colonoscopy, which is presented in a marvelously lucid manner with excellent illustrations. The various essential maneuvers are described perfectly. This is the best descriptive presentation I have ever read concerning colonoscopy.

The author then proceeds in an orderly fashion, covering anesthesia, anal abscesses, anal fistula, anal fissure, and hemorrhoids. Numerous helpful hints are given concerning the various diagnostic and therapeutic techniques he employs. The author is well recognized as an authority on the use of local anesthesia in anorectal surgery, and the technique described reflects his expertise. The chapter on pilonidal disease amply covers the management of this occasionally difficult entity for which so many procedures have been recommended.

The diagnosis and medical management of inflammatory bowel disease are taken up in great detail, and it is refreshing to have a surgeon write so knowledgeably about the medical management of colitis. This, of course, reflects the author's vast experience in treating the disease.

Polyps, diverticular disease, and cancer of the colon are presented in a thorough fashion. The chapter on cancer is of particular interest and especially informative. The pertinent comments made regarding technical factors in the surgical management of this disease are most helpful.

In summary, this book presents one person's considerable experience with the management of anorectal and colonic disease. It should be valuable to both the neophyte as well as the accomplished colorectal surgeon. I am most grateful to the author for the priviledge of sharing the writing of the foreword with such a distinguished surgeon as Dr. Beahrs. I would be amiss if I did not also thank Dr. Kratzer for the priviledge of having been taught all the information in this book by having been his first resident in colon and rectal surgery some thirty years age.

EUGENE P. SALVATI, M.D.

Foreword

Pathological conditions of the colon, rectum, and anus are most distressing, painful, and debilitating to the patient. When properly managed, relief is most often prompt, healing is permitted, and more extensive processes of inflammation and neoplasia are prevented. Although it is difficult to separate out minor from major conditions—those that might be treated in the office from those requiring hospitalization—most begin in stages that can be managed diagnostically and therapeutically in an out-patient setting. If a patient can be managed outside the hospital, there are benefits to the patient in convenience, time involved, and in costs.

It is most appropriate and timely that Dr. Kratzer has written a book on office practice in the treatment of disease of the large bowel. The content is based on his knowledge and experience of a professional lifetime as a fully qualified and expert colon and rectal surgeon.

Most appropriately the embryology, histology and anatomy of this part of the alimentary tract is first addressed since only if this basic knowledge is known can disease processes be fully understood. Diagnostic procedures are described, and indications for their use discussed. The approach to the patient is mentioned and this is most important since the disease processes are often painful and the examinations often lead to further distress. Successful evaluation and treatment requires the understanding and cooperation of the patient and good rapport between patient and doctor.

Anesthesia in the office for diagnostic and therapeutic procedures is addressed and most appropriately so since relief of discomfort permits a more careful examination and makes possible the management of many conditions which otherwise might require hospitalization.

Office management of common conditions of the anal region—abscesses fistulae, fissures, hemorrhoids, and other anorectal disease—is covered as well as the treatment of other local manifestations of more diffuse rectal and colon disease. Although the management of some of these conditions and especially their complications will require hospitalization, diagnostic medical, and minor surgical management can be carried out in the office.

Polyps of the rectum and colon are precancerous lesions and removal of these is a preventative measure against the development of cancer. Certainly, any physicians' office is a cancer screening and preventive facility and Dr. Kratzer has appropriately stressed the office management of these lesions.

To make the book a comprehensive document on colon, rectum, and anal disease, other conditions which are not necessarily office problems are briefly discussed since these are seen in the office but not always treated there.

The author has brought together under one cover the best of the state of the art in diagnosis and treatment of all abnormal and pathological conditions of the lower part of the alimentary tract emphasizing office practice. It is well done based on the wealth of knowledge and experience of an outstanding expert in colon, rectal, and anal disease.

OLIVER H. BEAHRS, M.D.

Preface

Perhaps more emphasis should be placed on the words "office procedures in colon and rectal disease." Since practically all patients are first seen by the physician in the office and many are treated there, a book on this subject is timely. Those engaged in family practice should find it particularly useful. Convenience to the patient and cost control are factors that are gradually making diagnosis and treatment of colon and rectal disease in a clinic or outpatient environment a necessity. Practically all diagnostic procedures, a majority of the minor surgical procedures, and most follow-up care can be performed as well, if not better, in an outpatient setting.

Most patients are relieved when told that they are not suffering from cancer and that their condition is an external thrombotic hemorrhoid, protruding internal hemorrhoid, fissure, fistula, pilonidal cyst or similar disease that can be managed as an office procedure. The fact that the patient can help make the decision in favor of outpatient surgery or other treatment encourages cooperation.

There are other factors that are making office procedures and a generally conservative approach to treatment more acceptable. Many patients, especially elderly ones, are apt to be suffering from more than one disease. Diabetes, arthritis, and cardiovascular disease may be present, and the anorectal condition may be the least pressing problem. Conservatism may therefore be in the best interest of the patient. In fact, even in the absence of other organic disease, there is a general trend to treat anorectal disease only if it is symptomatic. The experienced surgeon has always known this. There are many patients suffering from stress and tension who should be "talked out" of an operation unless it is for cancer. Often these patients will not only fail to be relieved by surgery but the condition may be made worse. This is especially true of patients with what are primarily medical conditions, such as spastic colon or idiopathic pruritis ani, in whom surgery might only add to their suffering.

Throughout the book, examples are drawn from my many years of clinical practice. I believe that illustrations are particularly useful in understanding the clinical principles important to successful office practices. I have therefore developed this book using a simple style, illustrating the procedures with detailed drawings and photographs. It is my hope that this volume will be useful to the medical student as well as to the more experienced physician.

Although the book emphasizes the more common colon and rectal diseases, the more rare conditions are also described so that there will be no difficulty in differential diagnosis. Follow-up of cancer patients in the office, for example, is written almost in "cookbook" style to avoid misinterpretations. Preventive medicine is given significant attention, since many colon and rectal diseases are due to poor diet, poor hygiene, and stress.

The intent of this book is to teach the physician how to diagnose all colon and rectal diseases, and how to prevent and treat most of them.

We find it impossible to list all the people who were helpful in the production of this book. Some provided the idea, others sustained the interest and many more helped to implement this project.

I owe a special debt of gratitude to the late Dr. Louis A. Buie, my former chief at the Mayo Clinic. I know of no one who has had a more profound effect upon anorectal surgery, and it is because of him that I have devoted my career to this discipline.

The chapter on colonoscopy is primarily the work of Doctor Asoo Kasumi, instructor in colonoscopy at Sacred Heart Hospital.

We reviewed the writings and accomplishments of men such as Doctors Robert W. Beart, Jr., Gerald Marks, Ira J. Kodner, A. W. Martin Marino, Jr., Bertram A. Portin and Eugene S. Sullivan.

Many others, including those writing the forewords or those referred to in the text deserve appreciation.

Miss Pamela Rauch, my correspondence secretary deserves much credit for repeatedly typing the original manuscript.

It was a pleasure working with Mr. Carroll Cann, Bob Butler, Carolyn Naylor, Joan Fraser and all of the people at the W. B. Saunders Company who produced the book.

My co-author, Mr. Robert J. Demarest and I have worked together on many projects throughout the years. Without his cooperation and patience, this book would not have been completed.

GUY L. KRATZER

Contents

CHAPTER 1

ANATOMY, HISTOLOGY, AND EMBRYOLOGY

INTRODUCTION

Since this book involves only office or outpatient procedures, it would be easy to describe only the anorectal anatomy. However, since examination and treatment of colon and rectal disease involves all structures from the distal ileum to the anus, other features, particularly as they relate to examination, are included. Sigmoidoscopy and colonoscopy with or without polypectomy or biopsy cannot be performed safely without an adequate knowledge of the related anatomy.

No two anal canals or colons are alike. Furthermore, surgical anatomy is significantly different from descriptive anatomy. The anatomy of the perianal area is best understood when palpation is correlated with visualization. This chapter will address only the principles of applied anatomy as they involve examination and treatment of colon and rectal disease. The reader is also referred to an atlas or textbook of anatomy, particularly for information concerning other than the pelvic structures. The 36th edition of *Gray's Anatomy* and Hollinshead's *Anatomy for Surgeons* are especially useful.

ANATOMY

Surgical anatomy should be accepted as an integral part of practice and, like all other patient considerations, must be approached gently. Inspection, palpation, and instrumentation constitute the proper order of approach to clinical examination, bearing in mind the normal anatomic variations that occur and differences between the anesthetized and the unanesthetized patient. We will begin this study with the perianal skin and describe the anatomic structures as they are encountered in examination, moving from the anal canal to the rectum (Figs. 1–1 to 1–3). The practical anatomy of the colon is included in the discussion of colonoscopy in Chapter 3.

The *anorectum* consists of the skin of the immediate perianal area, the anal canal, and the rectum. The skin of the perianal region differs from skin elsewhere on the body in that it is much thinner and has a finer texture. It

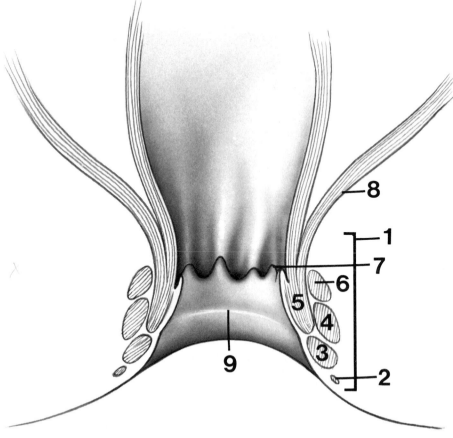

Figure 1–1. Surgical anal canal.

1, Indicates length of surgical anal canal.
2, Corrugator ani.
3, Subcutaneous external sphincter.
4, Superficial external sphincter.
5, Internal sphincter.
6, Deep external sphincter.
7, Dentate line.
8, Levator muscle.
9, Intersphincteric line (Hilton's white line).

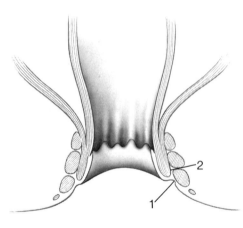

Figure 1–2. Relaxed anal canal.

1, Intersphincteric groove.
2, Internal sphincter muscle.

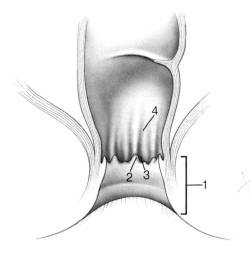

Figure 1–3. Anatomic anal canal.

1, Indicates length of anatomic anal canal.
2, Papilla.
3, Crypt of Morgagni.
4, Column of Morgagni.

contains sweat glands and hair follicles, both of which are absent in the anal canal. The external boundary of the anal canal is known as the *anal verge,* the transitional zone between the perianal skin and skin of the anal canal. The anus is not round, as generally thought, but is a slit-like or elliptically shaped opening surrounded by slightly puckered skin. The *corrugator cutis ani muscle,* a small circular band of smooth muscle not present in every individual, works in concert with the external anal sphincter to produce the slightly puckered appearance of the anus. This muscle, the most distal portion of the anal sphincter mechanism, surrounds the anal verge and is really a portion of the internal surface of the skin in this area. This band of muscle actually represents the ends of the conjoined longitudinal coat of the rectum (see p. 5). In very slender individuals, the contour of this tiny band of smooth muscle may be seen surrounding the anal verge.

Slightly higher in the anal canal, approximately midway between the anal verge and the dentate or anorectal line, a whitish groove may be observed or palpated. This structure is the *intersphincteric groove,* or inter-muscular ring. It is often more easily palpated than seen and is a distinct groove between the internal and external sphincter muscles.

The length of the anal canal averages from 1.5 to 3 cm in length when extended; its diameter is about 3 cm (Fig. 1–3). It begins at the anal verge, or the external margin. This external margin is a line formed by the walls of the anus as they come in contact with each other during their normal state of opposition. The internal boundary of the anal canal is at the dentate line and includes the anal crypts, or crypts of Morgagni. The *dentate line* is not a straight line but may be compared to a comb or saw with irregular teeth. It is a true mucocutaneous junction. Above the dentate line is the mucosa of the rectum and below it the skin of the anal canal. This line is formed in the embryo at 4 or 5 weeks when the cloacal membrane and anal plate disintegrate and, in so doing, leave a serrated margin. On the ectodermal side are small elevations of skin varying on the average of five to eight in number and known as the *anal papillae* (papillae of Morgagni). A modified transitional epithelium invests the anal papillae and their intervening free margins or *valves.* This same type of epithelium extends into and across the *anal crypts,* five or six small pockets or crypts at the dentate line with their openings superiorly. On the rectal side there are 6 to 10 *columns of Morgagni,* which are vertical folds of the mucosa.

The *internal sphincter muscle* is the lowermost, thickened portion of the smooth circular muscle of the rectum, which helps maintain continence. It is under involuntary control.

The external sphincter muscles and the levator muscles surround the surgical anal canal, which extends from the anal verge to the puborectalis (Fig. 1–4). The *external sphincter muscle* is under voluntary control, and is divided into three separate parts: subcutaneous, superficial, and deep. The subcutaneous portion of the external sphincter lies directly underneath the skin and just below the internal sphincter muscle; in fact, the interval between the internal sphincter muscle and the subcutaneous portion of the external sphincter muscle forms the intersphincteric groove, which can be readily palpated. The subcutaneous portion of the external sphincter is approximately 5 to 10 mm in diameter, although this varies among individuals. The superficial portion of the external sphincter muscle is elliptical in shape and acts as a sling on either side of the anal canal just superior to the subcutaneous portion of the external sphincter muscle. It is the largest portion of the external sphincter and the only part that is attached to bone. It arises from the tip of the coccyx, and after surrounding the rectum, some of the fibers may insert in the perineum body, although the greater portion of the fibers insert into the bulbocavernosus muscles (Fig. 1–5). This muscle contributes to the *anococcygeal ligament* or raphe. The deep portion of the external sphincter is primarily a circular muscle, although it tends to blend with the puborectalis muscle of the levator muscle group.

The *levator ani muscles*—the pubococcygeus, the puborectalis, and the iliococcygeus—are responsible for the strength and maintenance of proper position of the lower portion of the rectum and anal canal. The *puborectalis* is especially important to those interested in colon and rectal disease because of its direct contact with the rectum and its role in maintaining continence. Therefore, this muscle must always be considered during the surgical management of deep anal fistulas. The pubococcygeal fibers of the levator ani

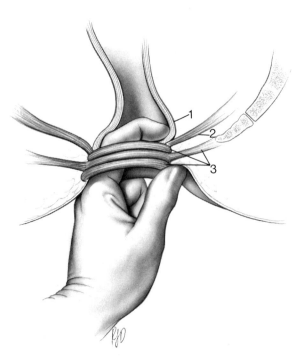

Figure 1–4. Sagittal section of surgical anal canal.

1, Internal sphincter muscle.
2, Levator muscle.
3, Three portions of external sphincter.

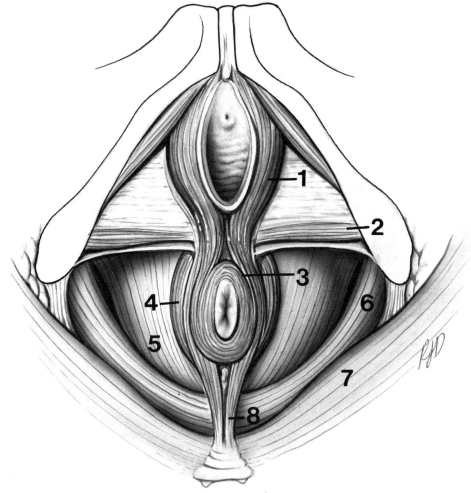

Figure 1–5. The perineum.

1, Bulbocavernosus muscle.
2, Transverse perineal muscle.
3, External sphincter muscle.
4, Puborectalis muscle.
5, Pubococcygeus muscle.
6, Iliococcygeus muscle.
7, Gluteus maximus muscle.
8, Anococcygeal ligament.

descend downward and fuse with the longitudinal muscle layer of the rectum to become the *conjoined longitudinal coat* of the anal canal. This conjoined coat passes between the internal and external sphincter muscles. It gives off multiple fibroelastic fibers, and some of these tendonous processes penetrate the lower portion of the internal sphincter mechanism and attach at the dentate line, thereby stabilizing the anal canal and preventing prolapse. Still other branches of this longitudinal tendon continue downward and through the lower portion of the external sphincter muscle to become the corrugator cutis ani muscle.

The *blood supply* of the rectum originates from the inferior mesenteric artery (Figs. 1–6 and 1–7). This artery continues to form the superior hemorrhoidal artery, which divides into left and right branches at approximately the third sacral vertebra. The middle hemorrhoidal arteries spring

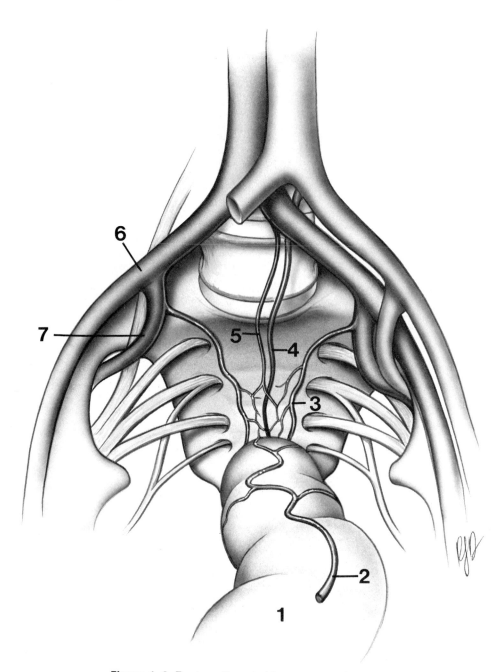

Figure 1–6. Rectum dissected from presacral space.

1, Rectum.
2, Cut end of superior hemorrhoidal artery.
3, Presacral venous plexus.
4, Middle sacral artery.
5, Middle sacral vein.
6, Common iliac vein.
7, Internal iliac (hypogastric) vein.

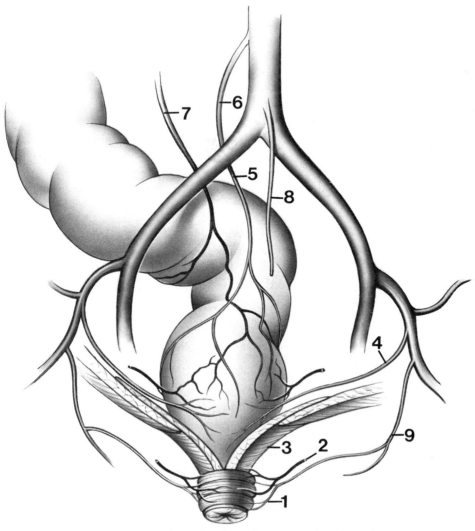

Figure 1-7. Posterior view of rectum and anal canal.

1, Inferior hemorrhoidal artery.
2, Inferior hemorrhoidal vein.
3, Levator muscle.
4, Middle hemorrhoidal artery.
5, Superior hemorrhoidal artery.
6, Inferior mesenteric artery.
7, Inferior hemorrhoidal vein.
8, Middle sacral artery.
9, Internal pudendal artery.

from the anterior divisions of the internal iliac arteries and proceed immediately along the lateral ligaments to reach the rectal wall, where they anastomose with the branches of the superior and inferior hemorrhoidal vessels. The inferior hemorrhoidal artery originates from the internal pudendal branch of the internal iliac artery. The artery leaves the internal pudendal branch, which lies enclosed in Alcock's canal, and runs medially and slightly forward, breaking up into branches that penetrate the external and internal anal sphincters and eventually reaching the submucosa and subcutaneous tissues of the anal canal.

The pudendal or *Alcock's canal,* a special sheath of fascia on the lateral wall of the ischiorectal fossa, is usually described as being formed by the splitting of the fascia on the obturator internus. This sheath or condensation of fascia, also known as the lunate fascia, begins posteriorly where the pudendal vessels and nerves enter the ischiorectal fossa and continues forward into its anterior recess, where the canal ends.

Undoubtedly, the main artery to the rectum is the superior hemorrhoidal, but it has been shown that after ligation of the superior hemorrhoidal and middle hemorrhoidal arteries, the entire rectum can survive having as its only source of blood supply the internal iliac artery via the inferior hemorrhoidal artery.

The *veins* of the rectum are comprised of the superior hemorrhoidal vein, which drains into the inferior mesenteric and portal system, and the middle and inferior hemorrhoidal veins, which enter the systemic venous circulation through the internal iliac veins.

The *lymphatics* of the rectum and anal canal follow the blood vessels supplying this part of the intestine, resulting in three main routes of lymphatic drainage: (1) upward through the lymphatic vessels and glands accompanying the superior hemorrhoidal and inferior mesenteric vessels to the aortic nodes; (2) laterally along the middle hemorrhoidal vessels to the internal iliac nodes on the corresponding side of the pelvis; and (3) downward through the pararectal lymph glands on the back of the rectum and along lymphatic plexuses in the anal and perianal skin, the anal sphincters, and ischiorectal fat to eventually reach the inguinal lymph nodes, which drain to the external iliac nodes.

The rectum has both a sympathetic and parasympathetic *nerve supply*. Of primary concern to the surgeon is the presacral or hypogastric nerve, which arises from three routes: a central one which descends over the bifurcation of the aorta from the aortic plexus and two lateral branches that are formed on each side by the junction of the lumbar splanchnic nerves and that cross the corresponding common internal iliac artery close to its origin. The aortic plexus contains preganglionic fibers that have descended from the thoracic splanchnic nerves through the celiac nerve.

The parasympathetic nerve supply is derived from small branches known as the nervi erigentes or fibers from the second, third and fourth sacral nerves on either side. The anal canal has both a motor and a sensory innervation. The internal sphincter muscle is supplied by the sympathetic and parasympathetic nerves, which presumably reach the muscle by the same route as that followed to the rectum. The sympathetic nerve is motor and the parasympathetic is inhibitory to the sphincter, serving to open and close the sphincter, respectively. The voluntarily contracting external sphincter has two sources of supply on either side, the inferior hemorrhoidal branches of the internal pudendal nerve and the perineal branch of the fourth sacral nerve. The levator ani muscles, which are a part of the voluntary mechanism of the anus, are supplied on their pelvic aspect by branches from the fourth sacral nerve and on their perineal aspect by the inferior hemorrhoidal branches of the internal pudendal nerves.

Although the word signifies straight, the rectum itself is anything but straight. It is S-shaped when viewed from the front and fits the concavity of the hollow of the sacrum when viewed from the side. The rectum measures approximately 16 cm in length. It extends from the dentate line to approximately the level of the second sacral vertebra. However, this varies considerably among individuals. When the rectum is straightened, as occurs during certain major operations, it becomes at least 10 cm longer. This occurrence is important in sphincter-preserving operations for cancer of the upper half of the rectum, since they require that sufficient normal rectum remain for anastomosis.

The rectum has no appendices epiploicae, haustra, or tenia, and is covered by the peritoneum only on its front and sides, while its lower portion lies entirely below the level of the peritoneal coat. The internal appearance of the rectum presents little of specific interest other than the transverse rectal folds or *valves of Houston*. These are permanent, sickle-shaped, horizontal folds consisting of mucosa, submucosa, and circular muscle that project into the lumen of the bowel. The valves help in temporary storage of stool in the rectum. Typically, there are three folds, the highest and lowest folds being on the left side.

Some confusion still exists concerning the *fascial attachments* of the rectum. On each side of the level of the second, third, and fourth sacral foramina, the connective tissue surrounding the paired branches of the superior rectal artery is attached to the sacrum and the parietal pelvic fascia by connective tissue that accompanies the middle rectal or middle hemorrhoidal artery and the associated nerves to the rectum. These tissues are known as the *rectal stalks*, or lateral ligaments of the rectum. There is also a posterior median attachment in the form of a strong band that passes from the anterior wall of the sacrum at the level of the third or fourth sacral vertebra to the posterior rectal wall. This is known as the *fascia of Waldeyer*. If the entire rectum is to be freed for removal, the rectal stalks must be severed between clamps and the posterior band must be interrupted by sharp dissection if necessary. Anterior to the rectal fascia, in the male there is a septum usually distinctly fibrous in structure that extends from the lower end of the pelvic peritoneum to the pelvic floor. This is the layer originally identified by Denonvilliers and commonly known either as *Denonvilliers' fascia* or as the anterior layer of Denonvilliers' fascia. This anatomic plane must be entered for easy separation of the rectum from the seminal vesicles and prostate, which is necessary in excision of the rectum.

HISTOPATHOLOGY OF THE ANAL DUCTS

The anal canal with a portion of the terminal part of the rectum and the attached perianal tissue was obtained from a male stillborn (8 months) at autopsy. All of the tissue was sectioned serially and the sections were stained with hematoxylin and eosin. From these sections it is easy to study the mucosa of the rectum, the skin of the terminal part of the anal canal, and that zone of transitional epithelium. The transition from mucosa to skin takes place in rather distinct steps. The first zone (zona columnaris) is the region of the rectal columns. In this zone the simple columnar epithelium of the rectum becomes two- or three-layered. The outer layer is simple columnar epithelium and the lower two or three layers are cuboidal epithelium. In the lower part of this zone (level of the crypts), the lining shows several layers of polygonal cells. The epithelium then gradually becomes multilayered and squamous (zona intermedia). Below this zone is true skin (zona cutanea), containing hair and sweat glands.

It is interesting to note that in this particular anal canal all the anal ducts show a lining consisting of polygonal cells, except one that shows a layer of simple columnar cells superimposed on a layer of cuboidal cells. In general, the lining of the ducts throughout their course is similar in that the cells are polygonal in shape and vary only in the number of layers. Usually the proximal part of the ducts shows a lining consisting of two or three layers, while the distal portion is composed of but one layer. The type of cell is certainly not unusual except that it is too low to be called columnar epithelium and too high to be called squamous epithelium. It is the type of cell that is seen in transitional epithelium.

In the specimen studied it is not difficult to visualize the course of these ducts. The course is not directly outward and downward, as usually described, but tortuous.

From detailed study of this anal canal it is possible to show that the ducts actually communicate with the crypts and penetrate the surrounding muscle (Figs. 1–8 to 1–13).

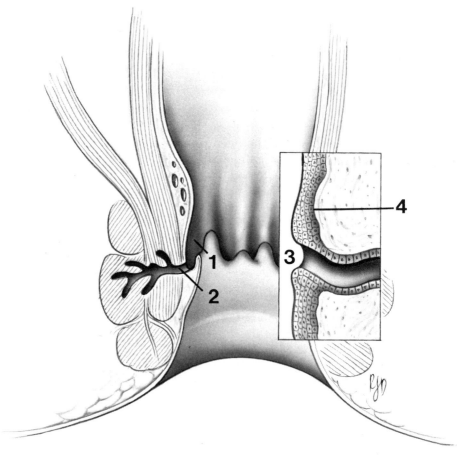

Figure 1–8. The anal ducts.

1, Anal crypt.
2, Anal duct penetrating internal sphincter muscle.
3, Entrance to anal duct.
4, Transitional epithelium.

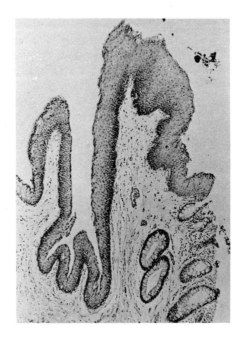

Figure 1–9. Normal crypt.

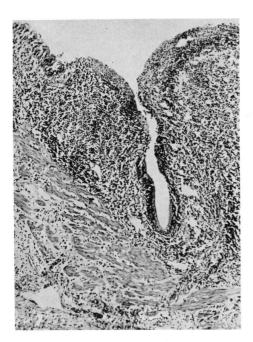

Figure 1–10. Cryptitis.

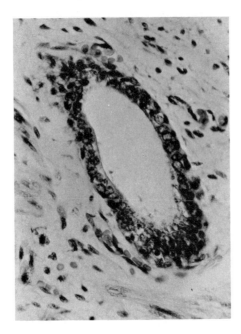

Figure 1–11. Normal duct.

Figure 1–12. Duct showing inflammation.

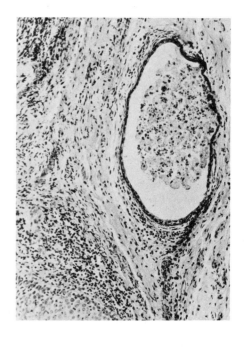

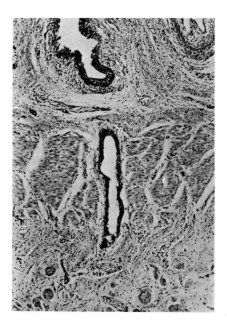

Figure 1–13. Duct penetrating the internal sphincter muscle.

REFERENCES

Hollinshead, W. H., Anatomy for Surgeons. Vol. 2: Thorax, Abdomen and Pelvis. Hoeber Medical Division, Harper & Row Publishers, New York, 1956.

Netter, F. H., ed., The Ciba Collection of Medical Illustrations. The Digestive System. Summit, N.J., 1962.

Williams, P. L., and Warwick, R., Gray's Anatomy, 36th ed., W. B. Saunders, Philadelphia, 1980.

2 CHAPTER

APPROACH TO THE PATIENT

HISTORY

The medical history is an important part of the diagnosis of colon and rectal disease, establishing the patient's confidence in the physician, and therefore making subsequent examination and treatment less difficult. A history of the patient's illness should be routinely taken. Remember that it is easy for the patient to generalize, and encourage the patient to be as specific as possible. Specifics such as the duration and character of the symptoms help establish an accurate diagnosis—for instance, an external thrombotic hemorrhoid has a sudden onset, while an abscess has a gradual onset. Be sure to cover the following areas: bowel habits (type of stools, presence of constipation or diarrhea), bleeding, discharge, distention and abdominal distress or anorectal pain, swelling, prolapse, tenesmus, and weight changes. All pertinent letters and reports of examinations from the referring physician should be obtained.

The general profile of the patient's physical and emotional status is also estimated. The art of office practice requires holistic as well as specialized knowledge. Most patients are under treatment for other problems, and it is important to know this before even a simple procedure such as excision of a thrombotic hemorrhoid is performed.

EXAMINATION

EXTERNAL INSPECTION

Always start with an examination of the abdomen. Check the general contour of the abdomen for masses, a distended bladder, or bowel obstruction. Let the patient point to the area of distress. Visible peristalsis may indicate obstruction, although in thin individuals this may be normal. Varying degrees of rigidity are an infallible sign of peritoneal irritation. Only the most gentle palpation is necessary to demonstrate this symptom; heavy palpation will only cause voluntary "guarding." Peritonitis may be localized or general, and it is helpful to determine this, particularly in treating diverticular disease. A spastic colon usually can be palpated as a tense, rope-like bowel. One must always be alert to the possibility of appendicitis or diverticulitis.

The abdominal findings may change or modify the remainder of the examination. Suspicion of acute diverticulitis would certainly make one proceed very cautiously with instrumentation, and appendicitis or a ruptured viscus requires immediate surgery.

Inspection of the anal area and surrounding structures is best performed in the knee-chest position, using the Ritter table, which is designed for this purpose. This position is also best for instrumentation other than colonoscopy. I find very little use for the left lateral (Sims') position, except for colonoscopy. Occasionally patients object to tilting the table. Good light such as that used in the operating room is essential to external inspection. The coccygeal area should be inspected. Sometimes tiny indentations representing minute sinuses in the skin of the posterior midline may be seen, which indicates potential pilonidal disease. Do not mistake the coccygeal dimple for this disease. After careful inspection of the coccygeal area, buttocks, and perineum, the buttocks are carefully separated to avoid any distress. Fissures, which usually occur in the posterior midline, may be detected by spreading the skin of the anal area. A skin tag may draw attention to a fissure. External hemorrhoids, protruding internal hemorrhoids, prolapse of mucosa, procidentia, papillae, or even polyps may be seen in this manner. On at least one occasion, I have seen cancer of the sigmoid present as a protrusion from the anus. Secondary openings of fistulas may be seen. The presence of a drop or two of pus at the anus helps to make a diagnosis of infection. Gonorrhea may present as a discharge of creamy pus. Sphincter spasm, atonic sphincter, or even pinworms may be detected in this manner. When in the inverted position on the Ritter table, some patients can relax the anal canal to such a degree that when the examiner gently spreads the anus, it is possible to see the entire canal and even the dentate or anorectal line, which marks the upper border of the anal canal.

DIGITAL EXAMINATION

There is no single examination that has more practical value than digital examination using the "educated" index finger. Most anal, rectal, rectovaginal septum, cul-de-sac, appendiceal, presacral, and even some gynecologic and urologic disease can be detected through digital examination. The fine granular "feel" of ulcerative colitis, the hobnailed sensation of Crohn's disease of the rectum, and occasionally aneurysms can be felt in this way. A soft benign polyp can be differentiated from the firm, cauliflower-like mass of a cancer. Even the enlarged, firm, harmless anal papillae that occur at the dentate line can be palpated. The digital examination also provides valuable information regarding the size of the anal canal and the caliber of instruments that should be used in internal inspection. The anxiety level of the patient can also be evaluated by noting the voluntary and involuntary activity of the sphincter muscles.

An extremely painful fissure with anal contraction may require modification of the usual digital examination by using the ring finger. The use of anesthetic lubricants or even local anesthesia may be necessary. In these cases I prefer to eliminate the possibility of colitis—which might be a contraindication to anorectal surgery—by performing proctosigmoidoscopy before excising the fissure or performing other definitive surgery such as partial lateral internal sphincterotomy.

INTERNAL INSPECTION

Much interest has attended the introduction of the flexible fiberoptic sigmoidoscope; however, in everyday office practice all that is needed is the Buie proctosigmoidoscope, equipped with suction to remove smoke in case it is necessary to fulgurate a polyp. A metal suction tube to remove mucus and liquid stool is also available. Gentleness is the most important consideration in introducing the scope to its entire length of 24 centimeters. To allay the patient's anxiety, it is best to describe to the patient the various sensations to be expected as the scope passes from anal canal to lower sigmoid. The patient will first feel fullness and an urgent need to defecate, followed by abdominal distress produced by pressure at the rectosigmoid junction. The rectosigmoid is the most difficult area through which to pass the instrument and requires special care. At this stage of the examination I usually ask the patient questions as a diversionary tactic. After passing the rectosigmoid junction, it is good practice to congratulate the patient on his ability to relax. With a relaxed and trusting patient the rest of the examination is easy and takes only a few seconds.

It may be necessary to pause to fulgurate a polyp in the sigmoid or perform a biopsy. In this phase, the only voice in the room should be that of the examiner. Do not alarm the patient. Do the job and then explain the findings to the patient. Never ask the nurse for a biopsy forceps or a fulgurating tip—hand signals are sufficient. However, just before using fulguration you should tell the patient about the buzzing sound that he will hear. If the bowel is not completely clean, it is advisable to give an enema before proceeding with fulguration. A Fleet's enema or a similar preparation can easily be given in this position. If a lengthy bowel preparation is anticipated, it is best to have the patient return at another time. In many instances, especially when the polyp is small, the tip of the scope can be manipulated so as to "wall off" the lumen of the bowel and complete the fulguration even if there is stool elsewhere in the colon. It is of absolute importance to avoid an explosion of gases within the bowel lumen such as methane and hydrogen. Methane has a distinct odor, and when this is noted, even when the bowel is clean, it is important to stop and prepare the lower bowel before fulguration. This should be done at another visit.

As the scope is withdrawn the entire mucosa must be observed. It may be necessary to inflate the bowel with a little air. Be sure to study the shelf-like valves of the rectum and the lower posterior "blind spot" of the rectum for hidden lesions. One must study many normal mucosal patterns in order to appreciate what is abnormal; this is especially true in recognizing early colitis. Normal mucosa is moist, shiny, smooth, and transparent. One can see the tiny pink arterioles and blue venules and myriads of tiny normal lymph nodes in the submucosal plexus.

Before the scope is completely withdrawn, the anorectal area is studied. Internal hemorrhoids, which are very common, are situated just above the dentate line. They usually appear to be pink or red rather than the expected bluish color. They are clumps of varicosities of the superior hemorrhoidal plexus, but arterioles may frequently predominate. In fact, there is a type of hemorrhoid that Buie recognized as arterial. They are rare but can cause such severe anemia that transfusion is necessary. In such circumstances, surgery is mandatory. The anal crypts should be observed for any evidence of pus or a tuft of granulation that might indicate the primary opening of a fistula. The size of the papillae should be noted. With the scope withdrawn, the external hemorrhoids that are covered by skin can be evaluated. Hemorrhoids, both internal and external, should be graded according to size on a scale of 1 to 4 (see Chap. 8).

After completion of proctoscopy the Hirschman anoscope, which comes in various sizes and lengths, can be inserted. The large, or number 3, scope is the only one generally used for close examination if there is a suspicion of a fistula or other disease. The crypt hook, which can be made from any malleable probe, can be bent appropriately for examination of suspicious anal crypts. However, just because a crypt can be hooked or is even ½ inch in depth does not mean that it is diseased or signifies opening of a fistula. The Hirschman anoscope may also be used for treatment such as the application of rubber bands for ligation of internal hemorrhoids.

Enemas are no longer used prior to the initial internal examination. In fact, the stool remaining in the rectum can be used for hemocult and other tests. The patient should therefore not take a laxative before the examination. It is easier to deal with a few particles of solid stool than with liquid and soft stool.

Colonoscopy is the greatest advance in the diagnosis and treatment of colon disease in recent history, and is discussed separately in Chapter 3.

BIOPSY

Biopsy and other specific technics will be discussed in detail in the chapters dealing with specific diseases of the colon and rectum.

COLONOSCOPY

INTRODUCTION

Since the report of the success of the fiberoptic gastroscope in 1956, considerable effort has been expended in examination of the colon by application of this technology. The flexible fiberoptic colonoscope was first described in the United States by Turell in 1963 in an article in which a picture of the instrument was shown without discussion of technic. In 1966, Lemire reported the successful visualization of the left colon with a gastroduodenoscope. In the same year, Provenzale reported the successful introduction of a fiberscope to the cecum by an "end to end" oral intubation method, and in 1967 Torsole introduced a fiberscope to the transverse colon by a "rope way" oral intubation method. Both of these methods involved using the expelled thread to pull or push the scope through the colon in a retrograde fashion. Shortly thereafter, Overhold described his flexible sigmoidoscope and reported the successful examination of the sigmoid colon. In 1969, Fox reported the passage of a thin and flexible fiberscope to the transverse colon by using a "retrograde colonic" intubation method, but he admitted that the "end to end" oral intubation technic was necessary to introduce the scope to the cecum. Finally, in 1970, Dean and Shearman described their work with the fiberscope using an Olympus intrument. They emphasized the superiority of this instrument over the rigid sigmoidoscope but stated that they still found the introduction of the scope into the descending colon difficult.

In Japan, endoscopists have been making continuous significant advances in colonoscopy. The development of the gastrocamera by Sakita and his colleagues in 1953 encouraged advanced methods of examination. The gastrocamera was fully developed by 1960. In the early 1960s, the Hirshowitz fiberscopes were imported to Japan, and using this newly acquired technology, many endoscopists attempted to make better and more efficient instruments.

In 1965, the Japanese Endoscopy Society held the first symposium on colonoscopy, moderated by Matsunaga. At that symposium, Niwa reported his success in examining the sigmoid colon, and Ohshiba described his 27 per cent success rate in introducing a colonoscope into the descending colon. Matsunaga and Kanazawa also reported the successful introduction of a scope into the descending colon in 59 per cent of their cases by using a special method involving the initial insertion of a polyethylene tube as a guide for the colonoscope.

In these early days, the introduction of the colonoscope was a difficult maneuver for many endoscopists. To overcome these difficulties, a new type of endoscope was designed. By the beginning of 1969, the colonoscope had developed into an instrument that is very similar to the one currently in use. In terms of the historical development of new endoscopes, endoscopists may be divided into three groups. The first group of endoscopists (Niwa et al.) developed the sigmoidoscope. Although the sigmoidoscope is short and can be used to examine only the descending colon, these physicians believed this length of scope was sufficient, because over 60 per cent of colon cancers originated in the rectosigmoid colon, and the examination of the rest of the colon by x-ray was not difficult.

The second group relied upon a special instrument with an overtube to overcome the sigmoidodescending junction (Matsunaga et al.; Fox) or tried to introduce the colonoscope by using the "rope way" oral intubation method (Provenzale et al.; Torsole et al.; Hiratsuka; Nagasako et al.).

The third group pursued the direct introduction procedure, anticipating future technical developments which would overcome the problems caused by the configuration of the colon. The persistence of the third group was eventually rewarded by the development of the alpha loop technic, clearly the most significant advance in colonoscopy.

In early 1969, after studying x-rays of colonoscopies, Tajima and Matsunaga discovered that in many successful colonoscopic examinations, the sigmoid colon assumed a shape like the Greek letter *alpha*. They used this observation and began to apply a torque to the flexible fiberoptic tube in situations where the sigmoid colon was N-shaped (a more descriptive term than "reversed S"). This gentle, counterclockwise torquing force, called the alpha loop maneuver, causes a temporary change in the configuration of the colon (Fig. 3–1). Establishing the alpha loop facilitates the introduction of the scope through the sigmoid into the descending colon. This maneuver eliminates the sharp bend at the sigmoidodescending junction, which is the major cause of failure to introduce the scope further at this point. Makiishi in 1971 soon followed the development of the alpha loop maneuver with a straightening maneuver that resolved the alpha loop into a straighter pathway (Fig. 3–1*G*); his splinting device could then be inserted to sheath the scope and help keep the colon in its new straight configuration. With the advent of these discoveries, colonoscopists realized that they could safely manipulate the colon more freely than they had originally thought.

Another development that accelerated the present boom in colonoscopy was surgical endoscopy. Early in 1969, the first successful polypectomy through the fiberscope was reported by Tsuneoka using a snare device in the stomach. His report of 43 successful cases was the beginning of the current popularity of polypectomy, and his paper was the first to describe the introduction of surgical technics in flexible endoscopic procedures. The sizes of the stalks of the polyps removed were smaller than 1.0 cm, and no significant bleeding was observed as a result of the procedure. Shinya and Dehle in 1971 applied a cauterization to snare polypectomy, making safer and thereby further popularizing the procedure.

Colonoscopy has been improving constantly, and if the few remaining problems can be solved, the technic will be fully developed. It has been shown to be an excellent procedure for examination of the colon, and an expert may even use it as the procedure of choice. However, reports of complications and complaints of patients' discomfort still occur. To improve the present situation, more specialists trained by experienced endoscopists are needed.

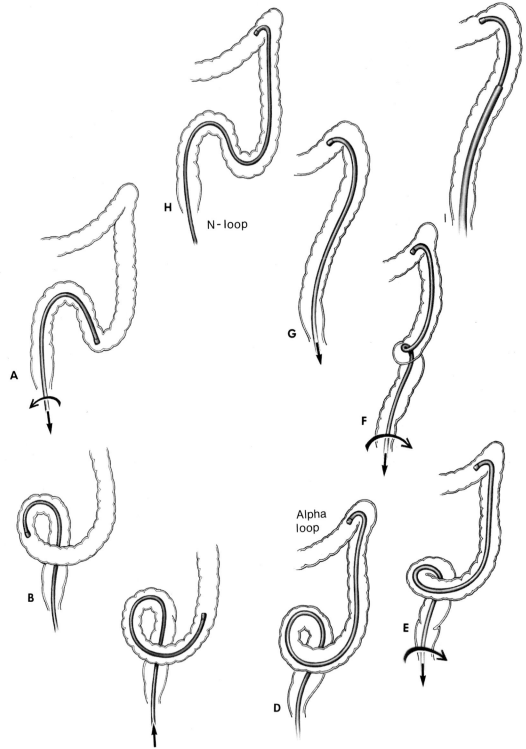

Figure 3–1. Alpha loop maneuver. *A,* Scope at the sigmoidodescending junction. *B,* Scope is turned 180°. *C,* Scope is inserted further to form alpha loop. *D,* Scope is introduced to the splenic flexure. *E* and *F,* Clockwise rotation and pull back of the scope will disengage the alpha loop. *G,* Straightening of the sigmoid results. *I,* Splinting tube is inserted to keep the sigmoid straight. If no splinting is used, the colon tends to revert to an alpha loop (*D*) or an N-loop (*H*), making further introduction difficult.

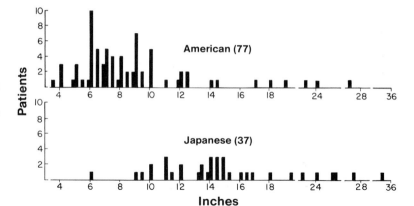

Figure 3–2. Variation in length of the sigmoid colon, American and Japanese patients.

The manipulations of a colonoscope that will ensure the successful introduction of the fiberscope in all patients is difficult because the configuration and length of the colon varies greatly in individuals (Figs. 3–2 and 3–3). Consequently, there is no one single method to follow. Technics that may be suitable for one patient may be totally inadequate for another. The technics used by acknowledged experts in the field also differ markedly. Tajima, advocator of the "two-man procedure," can reach the cecum within 10 minutes using the alpha loop method in Oriental patients, but it must be noted that these patients usually have a long colon with much inherent flexibility. Shinya, proponent of the "one-man procedure," uses the so-called shortening or straightening method on American patients. This technic is much different from Tajima's alpha loop method, but with it Shinya is also capable of reaching the cecum within 10 minutes with Caucasian patients, who characteristically have a shorter colon than Oriental patients. Although these two skilled endoscopists perform colonoscopy with different technics, the methods applied are obviously suited to the different types of patients involved.

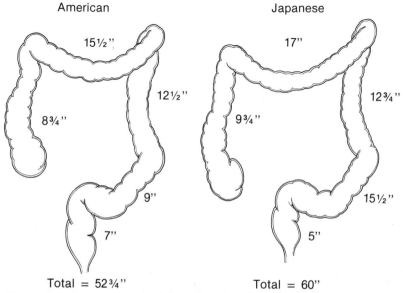

Figure 3–3. Average length of the colon, American and Japanese patients.

The history of colonoscopy is short in comparison to some other diagnostic methods. Therefore, it is understandable that the field is not yet completely established. As a result, some technics may not be suitable. In the following chapter, the basic technics and the "one-man method" of colonoscopy will be explained. The use of colonoscopy in diagnosis is discussed, where appropriate, in chapters on individual diseases.

General Considerations

Colonoscopy is a visual examination of the inside of the colon. To do this, one makes the colon change its shape to the ideal configuration of a question mark using the resistance of the colon, mesocolon, other abdominal organs, and abdominal wall as the support to advance the scope. The procedure does not consist of just simply following the lumen of the colon, which on many occasions would lead to difficulty. In a colonoscopic procedure, the tip of the scope must be advanced to the cecum, thereby ensuring that the entire length of the colon will be examined. This requirement necessitates the application of special manipulative technics to enable the quick insertion and advancement of the scope to the cecum while causing minimum discomfort to the patient.

Because the colon shows tremendous individual variations in length as well as in general configuration, no one pattern of movements may be suggested that will ensure successful insertion of the colonoscope; one must be adept at a variety of movements.

The motion of the instrument is limited but may be used advantageously to advance the scope. The scope may be moved in and out, or a clockwise or counterclockwise torque may be applied. The tip of the scope (an 11-cm portion at the end of the tube) is capable of up or down and right or left motions. A combination of these two motions may be used simultaneously to advance the scope. Obvious difficulties will be encountered in the regions of bends and turns in the colon, and synchronous movements of the tip of the scope and careful linear force or torque on the shaft must be applied to move the scope through these areas of changing direction. The physician must be careful not to distend the mesocolon or peritoneum and thereby cause the patient pain. One must utilize these organs to change the direction of the insertion power and make the tip move with minimal discomfort. The wall of the colon is thin, and care must be taken to ensure that it is not damaged.

These manual means of advancing the scope may be augmented by the use of suction. Suction results in a localized contraction of the colon in the region of the tip of the scope and causes the scope to be pulled further into the colon. Its application is most frequently used to assist the advance of the scope through the ascending colon; it may also be used to advantage at the splenic flexure and the rectosigmoid junction if advance by manual means is difficult.

THE ONE-MAN PROCEDURE FOR COLONOSCOPY

When colonoscopy was first developed, the fiberscope was short (about 60 cm) and was only inserted into the sigmoid colon. The insertion and examination could easily be accomplished by a physician working alone. Upon the development of the long colonoscope (180 cm), which is capable of reaching the cecum, the two-man method of colonoscopy became popular because of the difficulty for one physician to handle the insertion and advancement of the flexible tube while simultaneously manipulating the control unit. Because of their experience at that time, physicians were also concerned that they would lose their orientation, because of mechanical problems of the angle system, or that the manipulation of the tip of the scope and insertion of the scope would become difficult if the flexible scope was allowed to droop from the table or if it were wound upon the table. The technic that developed from these concerns involved the physician handling the control unit and directing an assistant to advance or retract the flexible shaft while the shaft is put straight. This is the original two-man method, which works well when the patient has a long colon and the distention method is applied. However, difficulties are encountered if the patient has a short colon, since the delicate shortening maneuvers cannot be done with this method. What is described in this chapter is a method by which a physician working alone can more successfully undertake the colonoscopic examination.

The major difficulty encountered by a physician attempting a colonoscopy without an assistant lies in the ability of the individual to coordinate both hands—the left hand to manipulate the controls of the eyepiece unit and the right hand to insert the shaft (Fig. 3–4). Once the scope has been inserted in the colon, the physician must not take his right hand from the shaft. Because of the nature of the torques and in-and-out motions used to advance the scope, the fiberoptic tube is rarely in a stable situation, and removing one hand from the shaft could cause the scope to move in an uncontrolled fashion. Consequently, all of the control features on the eyepiece unit must be adeptly manipulated with only one hand. Therefore, one must learn from the outset how to manipulate the controls with one hand, leaving the other hand constantly in control of the shaft of the fiberscope. This method in my opinion is superior to any other in situations in which the patient's colon is short or when the straightening method is used.

Preliminary Directions

How to Hold the Scope

In the one-man procedure, this is essential. Figure 3–4 shows how to hold the scope with the left hand. Holding the scope correctly is as important in colonoscopy as the proper grip is in golf. With the third, fourth, and fifth fingers and the metacarpophalangeal joint of the palm, grasp the scope tightly. The thumb must be completely free to turn the gears that control the up-down and left-right motion of the tip of the scope. Use the index finger for the suction and air buttons. Hold the shaft of the scope with the right hand, as illustrated in Figure 3–5. Use the right hand to introduce the scope, to pull or push the shaft, and to turn it clockwise or counterclockwise. With the right hand providing the power and the left hand controlling the angle of the tip, the scope can be advanced with gentleness.

Becoming Familiar with the Scope

To develop a feeling for the force that can be safely applied, place the tip of the scope against your skin and push it. When you begin to feel pain, that corresponds to the maximum force you can use. Memorize the extent of force you can exert, and never exceed this degree within the colon.

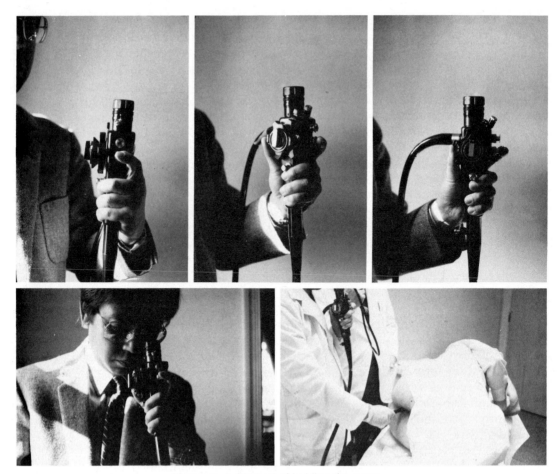

Figure 3–4. Method of holding the scope.

Air insufflation is often used to inflate a portion of the colon. How much air can the colon safely tolerate? The maximum amount of air comfortably tolerated is between 500 to 800 ml. Most fiberoptic scopes eject air at the rate of 80 to 100 ml/second. Depending upon the ability of the particular scope and light source you are working with, about a 10-second burst will provide all the air necessary to inflate the entire colon.

How to Practice the One-Man Procedure

To become accustomed to manipulating the scope, one must practice all maneuvers until they become second nature. Practice with one hand on the control piece and the other hand on the shaft, and watch constantly through the eyepiece. An easy and useful way to practice is by simply maneuvering the scope along a table top. Models of the colon are available, and practice with them will help refine the technic.

Care of the Instrument Before and After the Examination

The preparation of the instrument prior to an examination and thorough cleaning of the instrument after an examination are essential. The physician should examine the scope carefully before the procedure is begun. Even if you have cleaned it thoroughly after the previous examination, always check

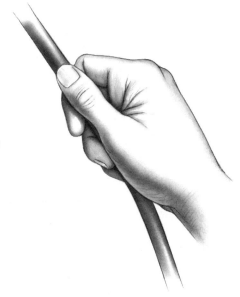

Figure 3–5. Firm hold of the shaft of the scope by right hand.

it before you begin another procedure. There is nothing you can do if you realize the scope is not working once you have begun an examination other than to withdraw the scope. This needless waste of time for both you and the patient can be eliminated if you simply check all the functions of the scope before you begin.

It is likewise extremely important to clean the scope thoroughly after completing each procedure. Part of a thorough cleaning is the disinfection of the scope.

An Analogy to the Colonoscopy Procedure

According to Shinya, colonoscopy is similar to driving a car. Just as anticipating a turn makes steering a car efficient and safe, keeping the car on the road, anticipating a bend in the colon avoids irritation by keeping the tip away from the wall of the colon. Of course, the added difficulty in colonoscopy is that the colon is constantly moving.

Review After the Procedure is Completed

To improve one's skill at colonoscopy, it is necessary to evaluate performance immediately after completing an examination. Mentally review the manipulations that were efficient; discard those that had no positive result.

The Importance of the Nurse and the Atmosphere of the Room

The importance of the role of the nurse or other assistant during the procedure and the pleasant atmosphere of the endoscopy room cannot be overemphasized. The nurse should be well trained and well acquainted with the procedure, and know how to help with any complications that may arise. The nurse should be cooperative, be enthusiastic about completing the examination correctly, and have true consideration for the well-being of the patient. The examination room should be simple and orderly. Quiet background music may help the patient to relax.

Premedication

Premedication with Valium (5 mg) and Demerol (50 mg) is suitable. Side effects accompany too much medication and decrease the patient's response to pain. The overmedication of a patient is actually dangerous, because the physician must rely upon the continual responses of the patient to the various manipulations. Some physicians oppose premedication because the colon may relax too much and thereby make the introduction of the scope more difficult. Premedication also requires time as well as a place for the patient to recover.

Opinions also differ on the value of administering an antispasmodic agent. Some physicians believe that some spasm of the colon helps to straighten the colon and aids in the introduction of the scope. It has not been my personal observation that spasm is advantageous in this fashion. However, in cases in which the colon is too spastic, medication with glucagon or another antispasmodic agent may be of help.

Technic of Colonoscopy

First and foremost, you must know the three-dimensional anatomy of the colon (Fig. 3–6). You should also be aware of the embryology, normal anatomy, and anomalies of the colon. Be constantly aware of the tremendous range of individual variations possible for the normal colon. Because of this range of configurations, the principal policy to follow while performing a colonoscopy is to try one maneuver only a few times. Do not use an unsuccessful maneuver repeatedly. If it fails to advance the scope or causes pain, try another maneuver. Progress from the easiest maneuvers to the more difficult ones.

The basic technic of colonoscopy consists of pulling back and searching for the lumen whenever encountering a near view of the bowel wall or loss of a proper view of the lumen. By pulling back frequently, the colon tends to

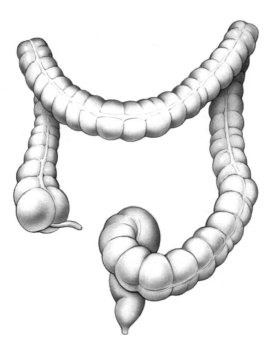

Figure 3–6. Three-dimensional view of the colon.

Table 3–1. IMPORTANT PRINCIPLES OF COLONOSCOPY

1. Watch the patient and assess his condition with every movement of the scope.

2. Once the procedure has begun, do not remove your eye from the eyepiece. View the interior of the colon constantly.

3. Always be alert to find out the center of the lumen and adjust the tip to it.

4. Do not bend the scope acutely when inserting it.

5. When advancing the scope, recall the pathway it followed upon entering the colon; think of the shape of this pathway when further introducing the scope.

6. Remember always that advancement of the scope does not rely solely on pushing the scope, but rather on a combination of pushing forward and pulling back.

7. Your right hand should firmly grasp the shaft of the scope at all times; never release the scope unless you are positive that it is in an absolutely stable position.

8. Remember that pain is a warning sign. Do not persist in any maneuvers that cause the patient pain.

9. Do the procedure as rapidly as possible to avoid irritation of the colon and the patient.

10. Be aware of your own abilities and know when to stop the examination and withdraw the scope.

straighten itself and is pulled towards the scope. It is best not to push the colon away.

Use the resistance of the colon, mesocolon, or abdominal wall to change direction of the scope while staying well within the patient's threshold of pain.

When inflating the colon, use the smallest amount of air necessary for examination.

Your success all depends upon your ability to find the lumen, to adjust the tip to it, to know and feel whether the scope is straightened or not.

Table 3–1 summarizes important principles of the one-man procedure for colonoscopic examination.

THE ANUS

It is not difficult to insert today's direct-view instrument into the anus, unless one uses the type of scope that has a wide hood. Before the examination, the anus should be well lubricated, and with the patient in the Sims' position, the scope may be introduced smoothly into the anal canal while under direct observation. Entry is facilitated by air insufflation to widen the anal canal. If the patient has a narrow anal canal, it may also be helpful to introduce the scope along a slightly oblique pathway (Fig. 3–7). Many physicians cannot find the lumen after a blind introduction of the scope. The examination may quickly become complicated by moving the tip of the scope in an effort to locate the lumen and thereby irritating the rectum in the early stages of the procedure. As long as you introduce the scope under direct observation, you should never experience this problem. If you lose the lumen at this stage of the examination, inflate the colon slightly, pull the scope backward a small amount, and the lumen should become visible. You may then make directional adjustments and advance the scope. In this context, lumen refers to the center or axis of the pathway through the colon, as shown in Figure 3–8. The importance of constantly observing the lumen cannot be overemphasized. Once the pathway is lost, minutes could be spent irritating the colon in an effort to locate the lumen again.

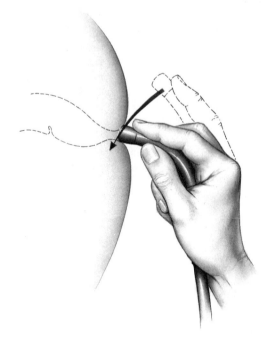

Figure 3–7. Oblique introduction of the scope into the anus.

Figure 3–8. A, Proper position in lumen. B, Improper position in lumen.

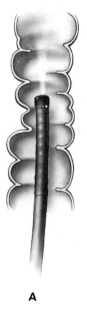

A

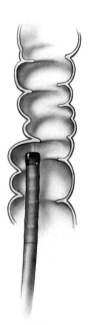

B

THE RECTUM

The rectum has a wide lumen and prominent valves. There should be no difficulty maneuvering the scope in the rectal area. After passing the rectal valves, the rectosigmoid junction is encountered.

THE RECTOSIGMOID JUNCTION

This is the first difficult section to pass through. Early attempts to pass this angle with the scope of less bending angle resulted in a maneuver known as the "slide-by" technic. The "slide-by" should not be used except in very special cases because it consists of a blind and dangerous introduction of the scope. The angle of the rectosigmoid junction can be passed easily in 50 per cent of the cases by adjusting the tip of the scope to the center of the lumen and proceeding. If the angle is sharper than the maximum angle of the tip of the scope, hook the tip of the scope to the bend and pull back gently. This area of the colon is not fixed, and by doing this, you can straighten the angle and thereby view the lumen of the sigmoid. Simply adjust the tip of the scope to the observed pathway and continue. If you still cannot introduce the scope, torque the scope clockwise or counterclockwise, and if you still cannot see the lumen, try the distention method; adjust the scope to the center of the lumen and advance. Then you can slowly see the lumen of the colon and can insert the scope. This will cause the colon to be lengthened (Fig. 3–9); then withdraw with a gentle, shaking motion and shorten the colon. Always shorten after distention.

THE SIGMOID COLON

From the rectosigmoid bend, carefully try to straighten the sigmoid colon after a few folds have been passed by simply pulling the scope back. Proceed slowly. If you take time to straighten the sigmoid here, you will be rewarded, because by straightening this section, the most difficult angle (that of the sigmoidodescending junction) will be easier to pass. You may add a slight torque clockwise as you withdraw the scope, but simply pulling back usually gives good results. Note that it is not necessary to bend the tip back sharply when you retract the scope (Fig. 3–10); this is a dangerous move.

Remember that the abdominal cavity does not contain the colon alone but the small intestine and omentum as well. Consequently, a simple pull does not make much if any change in the position of the colon. If you intend to change the lay of the colon, pull the scope back and shake the shaft repeatedly. Even this maneuver does not guarantee that the position of the colon has been changed and straightened, because sometimes it is simply impossible to alter it.

THE SIGMOIDODESCENDING JUNCTION

The sigmoidodescending junction is the most difficult angle to pass. In the United States, approximately one third of patients have short sigmoid colons that can be passed rather easily if you follow the lumen. One third of the patients have a somewhat longer sigmoid, and certain manipulations may be necessary to pass through it successfully. The remaining one third of patients have a very long sigmoid colon, and in these cases special manipulations must definitely be applied.

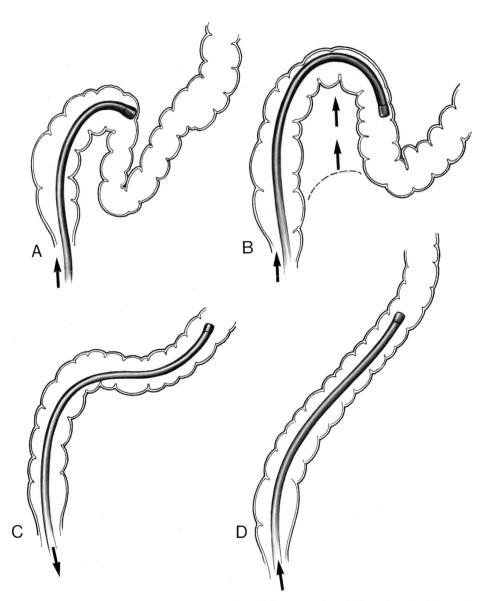

Figure 3–9. Lengthening and shortening of the rectosigmoid junction. *A,* Scope is introduced to lower sigmoid. *B,* Avoid making a loop. *C,* Scope is withdrawn. *D,* Scope is easily introduced after these maneuvers.

In a patient with a long sigmoid colon, if you attempt to continue the examination by just following the lumen, passage of the scope will become increasingly difficult. The pressure on the wall of the colon at the sigmoido-descending junction will cause the sigmoid loop to become larger and larger (Fig. 3–11) and ultimately will cause pain to the patient. This loop is called the N-loop. Difficulty in passing this loop is in direct portion to the size of the N configuration. Increasing force also causes the angle at the sigmoido-descending junction to become more acute, which makes passage of the scope more difficult. All maneuvers to pass this junction are attempts to make this angle less acute. To pass this angle, a straightening method must be used at the outset. To efficiently straighten the sigmoid, have the patient lie on the

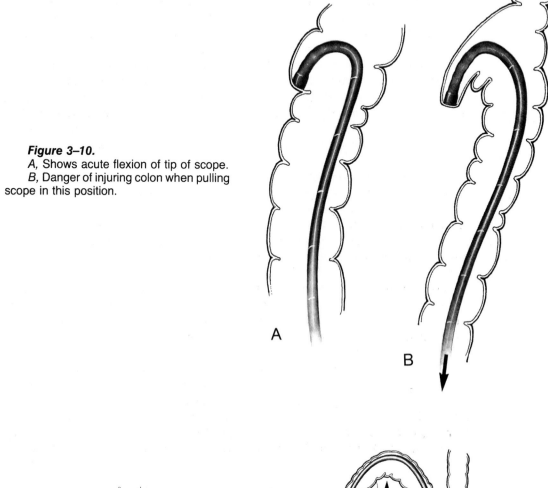

Figure 3–10.
A, Shows acute flexion of tip of scope.
B, Danger of injuring colon when pulling scope in this position.

A

B

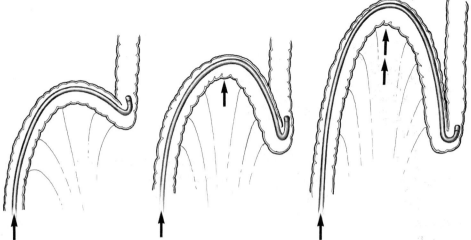

Figure 3–11. Difficulty in passing the N-loop.

left side to take advantage of gravity to straighten this portion of the colon. After the scope passes a few valves, pull back on the shaft while jiggling and shaking it to shorten and straighten the colon. An analogous motion is threading a long sock on a stick: You should not push too hard, or else the sock will just fold up on itself and not slip over the stick (Fig. 3–12). You have to shake the stick gently while advancing it slightly so that the sock may slip over it. While the task is more difficult with the colon because of the presence of other organs in the abdominal cavity, it is possible to change the lay of the colon by using this technic.

If the colon has been straightened to the sigmoidodescending junction, one can almost always pass the junction without undue difficulty. If the above-mentioned maneuver fails, however, one may try another maneuver to negotiate the N-loop. By following the lumen, the scope may be advanced to the descending colon, but a patient will usually experience pain due to tugging in the mesocolon (Fig. 3–13). Even if the tip of the scope is in the center of the lumen, pressure on the scope to advance it does not result in the forward progression of the scope but rather causes the stretching of the sigmoid colon and the regression of the tip of the scope (Fig. 3–14). This is called a paradoxical movement or a walking stick phenomenon. This phenomenon may also occur at the rectosigmoid junction, the splenic flexure, the mid-transverse colon, or the hepatic flexure (Fig. 3–15). To reduce this loop, advance the scope a little further than the sigmoidodescending junction, then carefully pull back. If the sigmoid colon is not too long, pulling back will simply reduce the N-loop and straighten the colon. Sometimes when you twist the scope clockwise or twist advance or pull back at this point, the scope may then actually advance further. This is called the "corkscrew" advance (Fig. 3–16). If the N-loop is very long, even if you hook the scope on a fold it may slide out when you pull the shaft back.

As an alternative to the above maneuver, the semi-alpha method may work for patients with relatively long colons that are not quite long enough for the alpha method. The basic idea is the same as the alpha loop maneuver but in this case, it is not necessary to make a true alpha shape of the colon to eliminate the sharp angle at the sigmoidodescending junction. After the shortening, corkscrew, and hook maneuvers have all failed, try to turn the

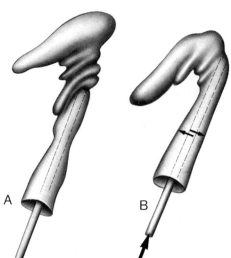

Figure 3–12. Analogy to threading a stocking over a stick.

A

B

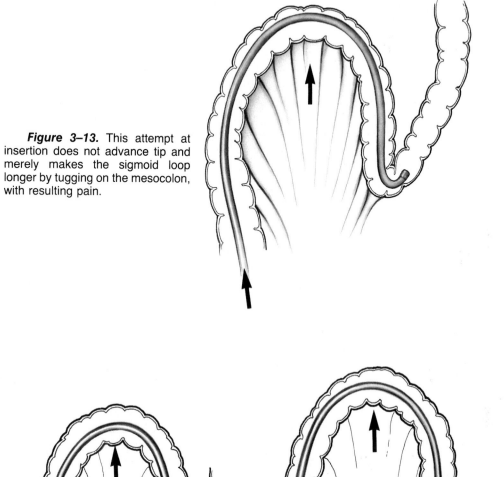

Figure 3–13. This attempt at insertion does not advance tip and merely makes the sigmoid loop longer by tugging on the mesocolon, with resulting pain.

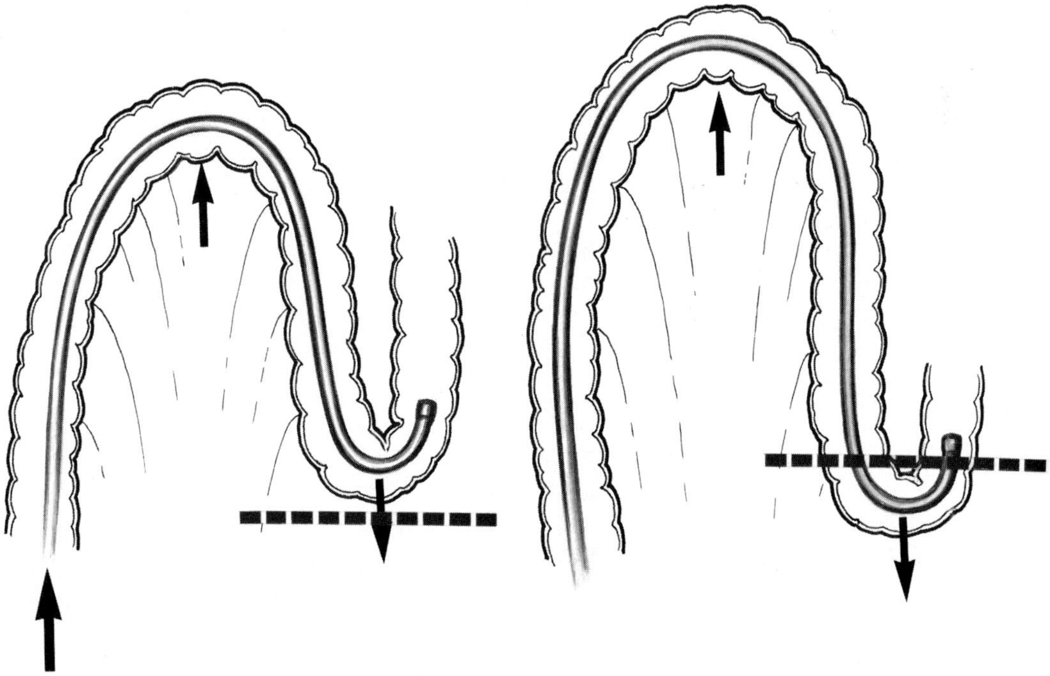

Figure 3–14. Walking stick phenomenon at sigmoidodescending junction.

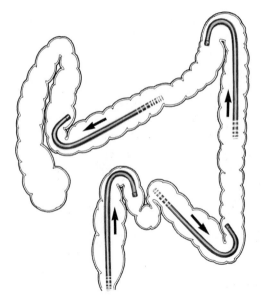

Figure 3-15. Walking stick phenomenon at other parts of the colon.

shaft counterclockwise, while jiggling and adjusting the tip toward the lumen. After a 180° to 360° turn, sharp angle of the junction will be lessened, the lumen will be opened, and the scope should pass through the sigmoidodescending junction easily (Fig. 3–17).

In the case of a very long sigmoid colon, the alpha loop may be the only maneuver that will work well. To perform the alpha loop maneuver in a patient with a very long sigmoid colon, while the tip of the scope is near the sigmoidodescending junction, turn the scope counterclockwise. Do not turn it if you feel any resistance or if the motion is painful to the patient. This motion eases the sharp angle of the sigmoidodescending junction, and the further introduction of the scope to the descending colon is facilitated. If the tip of the scope reaches around the splenic flexure, many patients begin to feel discomfort because of the increasing resistance to the scope, which in turn makes the alpha loop larger. This alpha loop should then be resolved by turning the scope clockwise and pulling back, which should straighten the sigmoid colon. After the sigmoid colon is straightened, a splinting tube may be needed to keep the sigmoid colon straight, because a long colon tends to revert to an N shape or an alpha loop whenever the scope is advanced further

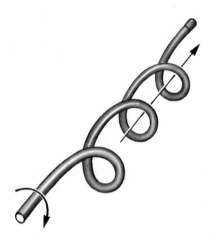

Figure 3-16. Corkscrew type of advancement.

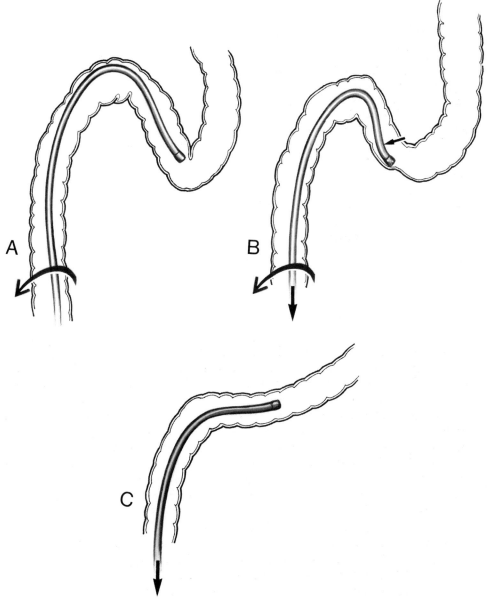

Figure 3–17. Semi-alpha method. At the sigmoidodescending junction, simple counterclockwise rotation (A) stretches the angle of the junction (B) and facilitates further introduction (C).

(see Fig. 3–1*I*). These particular maneuvers should be done under a fluoroscope, but even for regular office work you must know how to resolve this alpha loop because some colons naturally follow that pattern. Always be aware that the long sigmoid colon will tend to re-form a loop and that this tendency may cause difficulties when the splenic flexure, mid-transverse colon, and hepatic flexures are encountered. In these situations, application of pressure from the outside may be helpful (Fig. 3–18), or a splinting tube or splinting wire may be inserted.

If a splinting tube is used, it must be introduced under a fluoroscope.

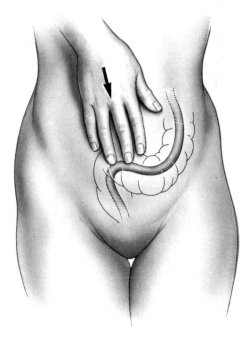

Figure 3-18. Outside splinting by hand.

Before the tube is introduced, the sigmoid colon must be straightened; whenever you feel resistance while inserting the splinting tube, do not insert it any further. Before this procedure is attempted you must check the surgical history of the patient for the possibility of adhesions and for any narrowing of the sigmoid colon. Either of these situations could be associated with problems in introducing the splinting tube. Splinting wire can also be used, but this approach is generally obsolete now. The wire can be introduced even in cases characterized by narrowing of the colon, but since the wire occupies the suction tube in the scope, one sacrifices the ability to withdraw air or fluid during the examination. In addition, the present type of wire is often not strong enough to keep the scope straight. If we can use a strong wire that withstands the pressure to bend the scope, then a special canal must be considered. I think this is the one of the solutions to make the ultimate colonoscope which has the changeable flexibility of the shaft like the one in Figure 3-19, with the help of special splinting wire.

The above-mentioned procedures are the principle technics that are applied at the sigmoidodescending junction. However, a different configuration of colon is occasionally encountered. For example, the alpha loop may be reversed, in which case the scope must be rotated counterclockwise to reduce the loop. Figure 3-20 shows other examples of complicated loops of the colon. The basic approach to the colonoscopic examination remains the same even in a complicated situation: shorten and straighten the colon whenever you can.

THE SPLENIC FLEXURE

After passing through the sigmoidodescending junction, it is usually not difficult to enter and pass the splenic flexure by simply following the lumen. Sometimes the lumen may be found behind a fold in the colon; by straightening the scope you may unfold this area and continue. If the patient has a high splenic flexure, you may experience some difficulty passing the scope

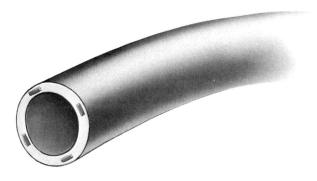

Figure 3–19. Fixed inside splinting device.

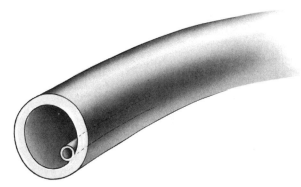

through it. Figure 3–21 shows how you may lower the flexure by hooking the instrument to the bend and pulling back gently to open the sharp angle. You can also accomplish this lowering by changing the patient's position (Fig. 3–22). The recurring problem in this section and in the rest of the colon is the tendency of the sigmoid colon to loop and curve whenever some resistance to advancement is felt at the tip of the scope. Pay constant attention to the sigmoid colon throughout the procedure, and be ready to use hands outside on the abdominal area to manipulate the colon, or splinting wire or a splinting tube to keep the sigmoid straight. This region may also show the walking stick phenomenon described earlier. The remedy is the same in this region of the colon: pull back gently to reduce the sharp bend and thereby enable the easier passage of the scope through this area. The presence of adhesions at the splenic flexure also may make it difficult to lower this part of the colon. In such situations, you must make doubly certain that the sigmoid colon is straight and gently pull back the splenic flexure as much as possible. Jiggling the shaft, turning the tip up and down, changing the patient's position, and using some suction may all be applied to advance the scope.

THE TRANSVERSE COLON

If no anomalies exist, you may simply follow the lumen through the transverse colon until the hepatic flexure is reached. A redundant transverse colon, however, causes specific problems that may result in the walking stick phenomenon at the mid-transverse colon. If the tip of the scope can be introduced a little beyond the bend of the mid-transverse colon, pulling back gently will cause the redundant colon to straighten and the tip of the scope to rebound and thereby move up and forward to the hepatic flexure (Fig. 3–23). You may also ask an assistant to hold the scope from outside the abdomen to prevent the scope from making the walking stick phenomenon

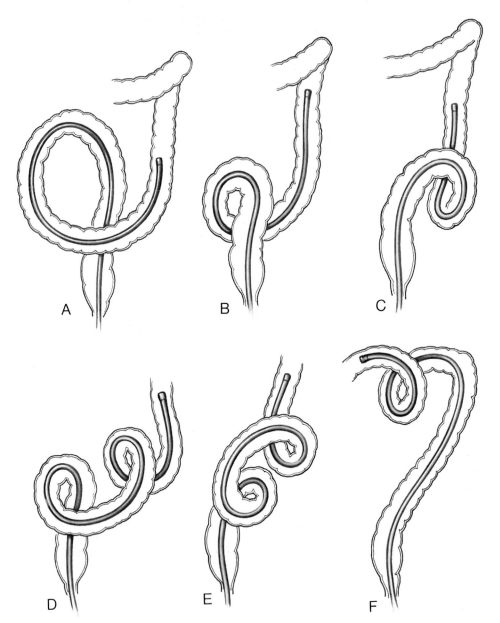

Figure 3–20. Abnormal loops: *A,* mega alpha; *B,* posterior alpha; *C,* reverse alpha; *D,* double alpha; *E,* double reverse alpha; *F,* gamma loop at the transverse colon;
Illustration continued on opposite page

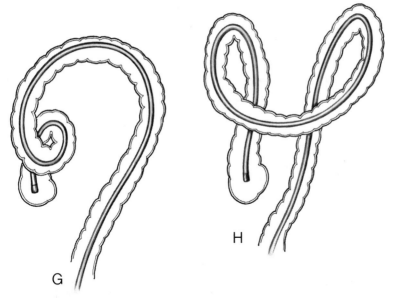

Figure 3–20. *Continued. G,* gamma loop at the hepatic flexure; *H,* two loops at the flexures. (From Sakai, Y., Eto, K., Mikaoka, M, et al., Abnormal loop encountered in colonoscopy. Gastroenterol. Endosc., 17:573–580, 1975.)

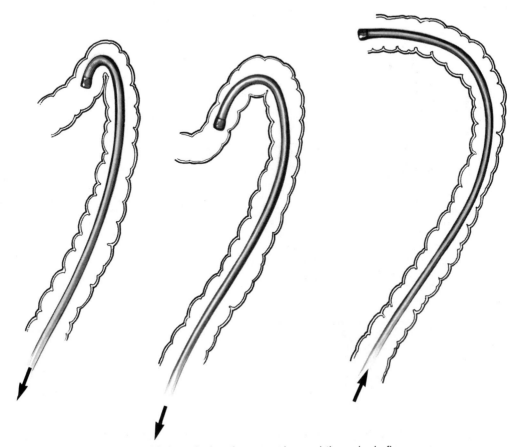

Figure 3–21. Introducing the scope beyond the splenic flexure.

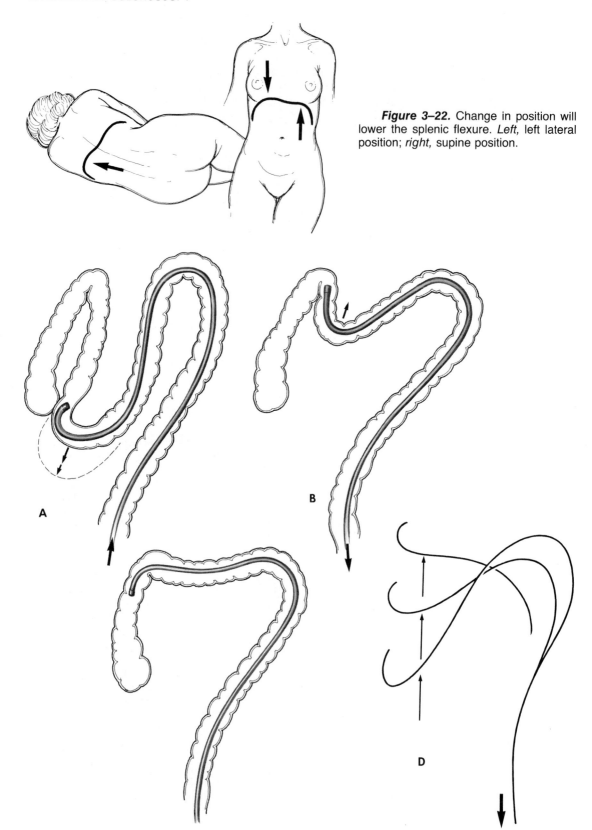

Figure 3–22. Change in position will lower the splenic flexure. *Left,* left lateral position; *right,* supine position.

Figure 3–23. *A,* Walking stick phenomenon at the mid-transverse colon. *B,* Pulling back on the scope brings the tip to the hepatic flexure. *C,* Scope is advanced to the ascending colon. *D,* Schematic drawing.

and going further down to the pelvic area. The transverse colon is located just beneath the abdominal wall; your assistant may actually hold the colon from the outside with his hand (Fig. 3–24). With the assistance of these two maneuvers, the hepatic flexure may be reached. If the transverse colon is very redundant, you may have to make a loop in this region intentionally by twisting the scope clockwise with the help of the outside hand and making an alpha turn. This procedure is rarely necessary in Caucasian patients.

THE HEPATIC FLEXURE

Once the hepatic flexure is reached, carefully look for the opening for the ascending colon. Do not try to advance if you cannot see the opening or the lumen. Occasionally, the opening is hidden behind a fold or is even tightly closed because of the sharp bend in the colon at this site. Search for it very carefully and never blindly introduce the tip of the scope. Once the hepatic flexure is passed, the shortening technique or deflation of air from the region or a combination of deflation and pulling back can cause the tip of the scope to advance deeply into the ascending colon.

THE ASCENDING COLON

Once the hepatic flexure is passed, the cecum can usually be reached without difficulty. In a difficult case you may be able to see but not reach the ileocecal valve. A careful combination of suction, jiggling the shaft, and the up and down motion of the tip of the scope will sometimes advance the instrument.

THE ILEOCECAL VALVE

When the scope has reached the cecum, pull it out to see the lower ascending colon, at which point you should be able to see clearly the cecum

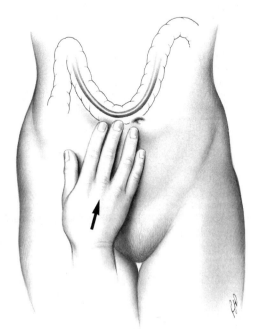

Figure 3–24. Assistant supports transverse colon from the outside.

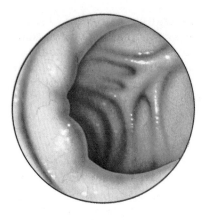

Figure 3–25. Ileocecal valve.

and the ileocecal valve. The ileocecal valve is usually on the left (at 10 o'clock), if the scope was introduced following a question mark pattern, or more rarely on the right (at 5 o'clock). Valves vary in size and shape, and may appear flat, slightly depressed, slightly elevated, flower-like, or donut-shaped. Usually you will only see a side view of the ileocecal valve (Fig. 3–25). Aim at the opening and introduce the scope just beyond the valve and bend the tip toward the slightly depressed area and cautiously search for an opening while gradually withdrawing the scope. When you see the opening, simply adjust the tip of the scope toward it and advance the scope. You should then see the terminal ileum. The terminal ileum has a velvety, villous appearance with scattered small lymphoid hyperplasia, and looks rather like the duodenum if there were no lymphoid hyperplasia. Usually it is not difficult to enter the terminal ileum, but in the case of a patient with lesions around the terminal ileum that need to be examined, entry may be difficult because the insertion to the terminal ileum still depends on the hooking method rather than the direct insertion.

Table 3–2 provides a summary of specific technics of colonoscopy, listed in the order of examination.

Indications and Contraindications

The indications and contraindications for colonoscopy should be decided on an individual basis. Although the trained specialist in colonoscopy finds it an easy, safe, and accurate method of examination, there are some situations in which it should not be performed.

The following are contraindications for colonoscopic examination:
1. Severe acute colitis.
2. Suspected perforation of the colon.
3. Recent abdominal surgery.
4. Impending perforation of abdominal aneurysm.
5. Recent myocardial infarction.

Office Colonoscopy and Polypectomy

There is no difference between colonoscopy done in an office and that performed in a hospital. Hospital colonoscopy is preferred in difficult cases that could be accompanied by complications. For example, the removal of a

Table 3–2. SUMMARY OF SPECIFIC COLONOSCOPIC TECHNICS

Anus
1. Introduce with air under direct observation
2. Oblique introduction may be best

Rectosigmoid junction
1. Follow the lumen
2. Use pulling back and straightening maneuvers
3. Distend carefully under direct observation
4. Always shorten after distention

Sigmoid colon
1. Shorten to facilitate passing the sigmoidodescending junction

Sigmoidodescending junction
1. Shortening from the beginning
2. Shortening after distention
3. Use a corkscrew maneuver
4. Hooking with the tip of the scope
5. Semi-alpha loop maneuver
6. Alpha loop maneuver

Splenic flexure
1. Straighten the sigmoid and follow the lumen
2. Lower the splenic flexure
3. Change position of patient

Transverse colon
1. Follow the lumen
2. Rebound method for scope advancement
3. Hold the scope from the outside

Hepatic flexure
1. Follow the lumen
2. Hook and pull

Ascending colon
1. Air suction and pulling back

Ileocecal valve
1. Introduce tip a little beyond valve
2. Bend and search for opening
3. Pull slowly aiming at the opening

Special manuevers to pass difficult places
1. Minimum air insufflation
2. Always adjust the tip to the center of the lumen
3. Make sure the scope is following the question mark shape
4. Air suction
5. Move the tip up and down or right and left
6. Jiggle the shaft
7. Move the scope continuously and look for the opportunity to insert quickly or gradually as indicated.

large polyp or the examination of a poor-risk patient may be best performed in a hospital, where an ER system is available. However, in normal cases the unfamiliar, impersonal atmosphere of a hospital may only serve to upset the patient and make the examination more difficult. While an ER system is not available, the familiar, relaxed atmosphere of an office provides a more suitable environment for colonoscopy. For polypectomy, one arbitrary designation, I consider sessile polyps of less than 1.5 cm in diameter and pedunculated polyps with a stalk of 0.7 cm or less in diameter as suitable for outpatient treatment.

PRECAUTIONS IN POLYPECTOMIES

The following are some precautions that should be taken if polypectomy is performed in the course of a colonoscopic examination. The diagnosis and management of polyps are discussed more fully in Chapter 13.

- Know the capabilities of the cauterization instrument and snare.
- Make sure that the cautery instrument is working before inserting the scope.
- Observe carefully whether the polyp is real. Hemangiomas, submucosal tumors, and inverted diverticula can be mistaken for polyps.
- Examine the entire colon prior to polypectomy.
- Decide in advance where to snare the polyp.
- Draw out the mucus around the polyp by using the suction of the scope and clean the base of the polyp. Use suction and inflation alternately to rid the area of any explosive gases if the colon is not really clean. Put the scope in the best position to perform the polypectomy.
- Distend the colon properly when snaring the polyp; do not include the adjacent mucosa.
- Make sure that the snare never touches the normal mucosa.
- Never snare a sessile polyp deeply nor prolong coagulation.
- If done properly, the mucosa should change to a white color when beginning coagulation and then gradually cut while current is being applied.
- If the polyp is large or the lumen narrow, it may be impossible to keep the head of the polyp from the colon wall during the polypectomy. Avoid long contact with the mucosa by oscillating the polyp during coagulation. In such instances, it is important to see definite whitening of the stalk, bearing in mind that the bulk of the current usually goes to the head of the polyp.
- Be aware that even if the polypectomy is performed well, bleeding can occur as long as 14 days after the procedure.

QUESTIONS AND ANSWERS

How many ways are there to perform colonoscopy?

There are four ways to perform a colonoscopic examination.

The original method is known as the two-man method. Because the colonoscopes were long compared with the gastroscope, manipulations of the instrument by one man were difficult. Also, the original idea of colonoscopy called for the flexible shaft to be kept straight. This practice made it easier for the operator to be aware of the tip of the scope and to make full use of the angle, which was not as manageable as in today's instruments. The second man was necessary to follow the examining physician's directives regarding the introduction of the scope. This is still considered a good procedure when a physician is dealing with a patient with a long colon, and many Japanese physicians perform this method excellently.

The so-called "reformed two-man method" is an outgrowth of the development of the teaching scope. With this instrument, two physicians can view the interior of the colon at the same time, and both doctors can manipulate the scope independently. Although occasionally this procedure can be done well if the two physicians cooperate and communicate clearly, most often the two are less efficient than one physician with a good assistant. This method is what is commonly referred to as the two-man method in current use.

The first "one-man method" has become popular. Because of improvements in the scope itself, most doctors are no longer worried about the lack of angulation of the shaft which can come from winding or bending of the scope. In this method, the doctor manipulates the shaft of the scope and the wheel that controls the left and right orientation of the tip of the scope with the right hand while the left hand moves the wheel that controls the up and down motion of the tip. This method works in a fashion very similar to the original two-man method, in that one cannot shorten the colon from the beginning of the procedure.

The second "one-man method" calls for the physician to manipulate all systems of the control piece with the left hand and the shaft of the scope with the right hand. It is especially important that the right hand always holds the shaft. This is the best style in which to hold the scope and in this fashion, one may shorten the colon from the very beginning of the procedure. The alpha loop maneuver and other procedures are accomplished without aid from an assistant or another physician. In this context, this is truly a "one-man method."

What is the value of premedication?

The success of the colonoscopic examination will probably rest on whether or not the patient can relax. The best way to approach this problem is to explain the importance of the examination to the patient and also to describe how easy it will be. Some doctors may show the instrument to the patient, but this may not be a good idea for every patient. All instruments should normally be hidden from the patient's view.

I usually use 5 mg of Valium and 50 mg of Demerol to help the patient to relax. There is some controversy about the value of premedication. More side effects occur from the injection of the medication than from the colonoscopic procedure itself. Premedication may also hinder or prevent the examination by causing too much relaxation of the colon. However, I prefer to give sedation, but only to the point of relaxing the patient sufficiently to ensure his comfort. Medication should not be used to compensate for poor technic.

How important is simple manual dexterity?

There is no other examination that more clearly reflects differences in manual dexterity among physicians than colonoscopy. The success of the examination depends solely upon whether the doctor can take the proper action and react to the changing situation of the colon throughout the procedure. The colon is constantly moving during the examination, and the physician must be prepared to respond to the motion and to follow the lumen as rapidly as possible. To perform the procedure well, the colonoscopist must master every technic of scope control.

How great are the anatomic differences among colons?

Few doctors realize that no other organ shows the vast individual variations that are typical of the colon (see Figs. 3–2 and 3–3). In addition to remarkable anatomic differences among colons, the same colon will show a different response to colonoscopy from day to day. This fact makes colonoscopy the most difficult procedure in the field of endoscopy.

The variability of anatomy and disposition of the colon is the major reason why no single procedure may be described that will advance the scope successfully every time. The examining physician must be constantly aware of the condition of the patient and immediately responsive to any pain the patient experiences. Again, it must be stressed that if a maneuver does not work, cease using it and try another.

Does the colon change from day to day?

The condition of the colon is different every day. If you cannot perform a colonoscopic examination one day, it may be much easier on the next day.

Consequently, rather than taking a long time on one day when the examination is not proceeding well, simply stop and try again another day.

What is the ideal way of inserting the scope?

Good colonoscopic technic requires that you do not simply follow the lumen but that you make the colon change its shape to the ideal configuration of a question mark. A combination of advancing the scope, pulling back, directing the scope to the lumen again and advancing, and then pulling back is the suggested way to accomplish this. Other maneuvers for different regions of the colon have been summarized in Table 3–2.

How important is the angle of the tip of the fiberoptic scope?

The modern fiberoptic scope has been improved by increasing the angle at which the tip of the scope may be bent. However, the sharpest possible angle is not always necessary in the colonoscopic procedure. If the tip of the scope is bent too much, the power used to introduce the scope is not transmitted to the tip but rather to the shaft of the scope immediately behind the tip. The result of this is the walking stick phenomenon, discussed previously. Whenever you are trying to insert the colonoscope, make sure that the scope has an angle at the tip that will enable its smooth and direct introduction through the lumen.

What use is the arrow visible through the scope on its tip?

The small triangular sign on the tip of the scope merely corresponds to the direction the tip will move when the "up" knob is twisted on the control unit. Obviously, when the "down" knob is twisted, the tip of the scope will move in the opposite direction. It is important to realize that because of the twisting and bending of the scope as it progresses through the colon, the movement does not correspond to "up" and "down" in any anatomic sense. If you wish to know the orientation within the colon, you may look at the water accumulated inside the colon. If there is no water, squirt a small amount in and observe where it rests. The water will always accumulate in the lowest part of the colon available to it, and you can use that fact to orient yourself.

Is there one single thing that makes flexible endoscopy so difficult?

The bends in the colon are the single feature that make colonoscopy so difficult. To complicate matters, you can form other bends without realizing it while advancing the scope (Fig. 3–26). The five naturally occurring bends in the colon are indicated in Figure 3–27. This is why the best way to insert the scope is to eliminate the bends by shortening and straightening whenever possible. The ideal shape for the colon to assume during a colonoscopic examination is that of a question mark, with all angles flat and smooth.

What is the importance of the pulling back maneuver?

The purpose of colonoscopy is to insert the scope to the cecum and enable the visual examination of the entire lumen. The idea of pulling the scope back sounds counterproductive, but the importance of this movement must be stressed. If the scope is not withdrawn a little bit after it has been advanced, you will be unable to see the lumen, you will be more likely to make an unwanted loop, and you will be more likely to introduce the scope blindly and risk perforating the colon. The important factor is not what length of scope has been inserted, but rather what extent of the colon has been passed through. Recall what was described in the section on "threading"

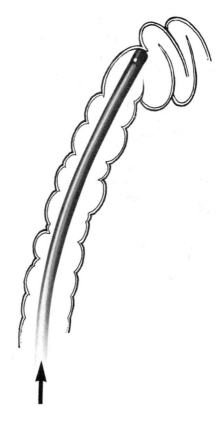

Figure 3–26. Loop made by careless introduction of scope.

the colon onto the shaft of the colonoscope, remember the tremendous expandability and flexibility of the colon, and you will understand the difference. I become concerned if I have introduced the scope over 80 cm without reaching the ascending colon. The splenic flexure is usually reached by 40 cm to 60 cm when the scope is straight. Inserting too much of the scope usually means that the colon has been extended and the patient is probably uncomfortable.

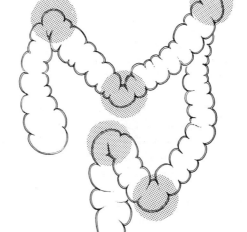

Figure 3–27. Normal angles of the colon.

What are shortening and straightening?

Shortening and straightening refer to those movements that flatten the angles in the difficult bends in the colon and thread the colon onto the flexible shaft of the scope. Of the two ways to accomplish these maneuvers, the first, shortening and straightening from the beginning of the examination, is preferable to the second, shortening and straightening only after distention.

To shorten and straighten the colon from the beginning of the examination, manipulate the shaft with the right hand, never removing the hand from the shaft throughout the procedure. After passing a few folds, pull the scope back slightly or apply a slight clockwise rotation and level the colon by jiggling the shaft of the scope. Remember that you are trying to change the lay of the colon amidst the other organs within the abdominal cavity. Shortening and straightening the colon from the beginning of the examination is the best technic to use for a patient with a short or intermediate-length colon. For a patient with a long colon, one has no other alternative than also to distend the colon, especially in the region of the sigmoid colon, and to shorten and straighten after distension.

Should one try an alpha loop maneuver on every patient?

The alpha loop method was developed by Japanese physicians and works very well on patients with long colons. Establishing an alpha loop should be done under the fluoroscope, as should straightening the loop and introducing a splinting tube. If the colon follows an alpha loop naturally, fluoroscopic visualization may not be necessary. The alpha loop is not always feasible on American patients, most likely because the anatomy of the colon in the sigmoidal region is different from that of Japanese patients. Not only the length of the sigmoid but also the length of the mesocolon in that region will influence the physician's ability to form an alpha loop. Because the length of the mesocolon cannot be evaluated from x-rays, simply looking at the length of the sigmoid colon in a radiograph may mislead a physician about the possibility of doing the alpha loop maneuver. As has been indicated before, of the one third of the American population that have long colons, the alpha loop maneuver will not only be possible but also necessary to insert the colonoscope successfully.

Are there alternatives to the alpha loop maneuver?

The alpha loop maneuver was devised for those patients with a long sigmoid colon and a long mesocolon; it facilitates the insertion of the colonoscope to the sigmoidodescending junction, which is characteristically sharply bent in these patients. For the patient with a short sigmoid colon and short mesocolon, creating the alpha loop may be dangerous. For these types of patients, a so-called semi-alpha loop is advocated. If a few attempts at shortening the colon at the sigmoidodescending junction fail, try to turn the scope counterclockwise. The colon may gradually change its position and introduction of the scope into the descending colon will then be easier. For short colons that cannot assume the alpha loop shape, the semi-alpha loop may provide an alternative maneuver to enable easier passage through the sigmoidodescending junction.

Can you form loops without knowing it?

Loops in the colon may form regardless of how one tries to avoid them. In principle, one should reduce these loops one by one and then proceed.

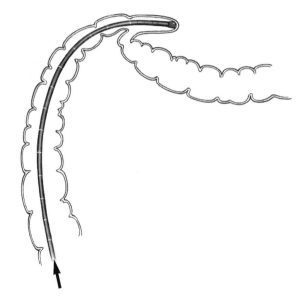

Figure 3–28. Possible error caused by "slide-by" technique.

What is the "slide-by" technic of scope advancement?

Before manufacturers of colonoscopes developed the highly flexible angle systems on the tips of modern scopes, the "slide-by" technic was applied to overcome the sharp angles of the colon. During this maneuver, the tip of the scope slides along the colon wall. As long as the instrument stays in the lumen, there are no problems, but if you look at the x-ray while doing the sliding, you will be surprised how much the tip deforms the colon wall (Fig. 3–28). The colon will be distended and the patient will feel pain. In addition, it is very easy to perforate the colon if the tip of the scope enters a blind pouch and continuous pressure is applied. Now that instrumentation has been improved, there is no need to attempt the slide-by technic. Remember that colonoscopy involves not just the introduction of the scope to the cecum by following the lumen, but implies that technics should be used to position the colon in its most favorable shape to accept the scope as rapidly as possible. The more rapidly the colon assumes the classic question-mark shape, the less the discomfort to the patient. Because the slide-by technic distends the colon needlessly, it should not be used.

How can you determine what portion of the colon the tip of the scope has reached?

1. If you are at a bend in the colon, you are most likely at:
   a. the rectosigmoid junction
   b. the sigmoidodescending junction
   c. the splenic flexure
   d. the mid-transverse colon
   e. the hepatic flexure
Then you can guess where you are by the length of the scope.
2. The transverse colon often has a triangular shape.
3. If the colon wall looks bluish, you may be at:
   a. the hepatic flexure
   b. the splenic flexure
   c. the sigmoidodescending junction
Again, you can guess where you are by length.

4. The ileocecal valve has the typical appearance shown in Figure 3–25, and the pouch of the cecum looks like a crow's foot.
5. Dark, watery stool content is often found in the right side of the colon.
6. Light can often be perceived through the abdominal wall, especially at the cecum or transverse colon.
7. If the tip of the scope is in the cecum, gentle tapping with the fingers on the ileocecal region can be noted inside the colon.
8. If you can be sure that the scope is straight and not looping, the length of the scope that has been introduced should serve as an indicator of the location of the tip within the colon. Always remember, however, that even if the scope is introduced to its 80-cm mark, the usual length to the cecum, the tip may be only at the sigmoidodescending junction because of looping.
9. X-ray examination is the best single method by which one can determine the location of the tip of the scope in the colon. Even with x-ray and with all other methods, do not rely on only one indicator but rather use two or three to determine the tip's location.

Are x-rays necessary?

A current troublesome trend in colonoscopy is to consider the endoscopist who can introduce the scope without concurrent radiographic examination a better endoscopist than one who uses x-rays. In one sense this may be true. An obvious advantage of colonoscopy is that the procedure does not require radiation. However, for the beginner and especially for the resident, it is almost impossible to perceive what is happening during a colonoscopic examination without the help of x-rays. The education of a colonoscopist must begin with a visual understanding of the process of inserting the scope through the colon. Understanding how the scope is inserted and how it may be made to progress through the colon is crucial to the successful completion of an examination. The consequence of failing to understand the three-dimensional architecture of the colon and how it changes during colonoscopy in response to manipulations of the scope is at the least useless pain for the patient and at worst perforation of the colon itself. In some cases, it is also very difficult to determine the location of the tip of the scope. While there are several internal physical features that help indicate the location of the tip of the scope (enumerated in the previous question), at times it is difficult even for an expert to pinpoint the location without x-rays.

What is meant by "proper air"?

Teaching endoscopy must include a discussion of the proper amount of air used to inflate the colon. This concept is critical, because a good view of the interior is impossible without proper air insufflation, and lesions may be missed without proper air to expand a region slightly. Caution is advised, however, for it is also possible to cause considerable discomfort or even a tear in the colon wall if too much air is used. A person learning endoscopy should know how much air per second the scope can eject and also how much air per second the scope can draw out. Some doctors believe that the modern colonoscopes have too powerful an air insufflation system, but weaker systems would require too much time to inflate the colon, thereby slowing down the examination. Again, if you know the capacity of your scope, providing proper air presents no difficulty or danger and enables a good and rapid examination.

What is the optical system of the fiberoptic scope?

Unfortunately, the actual number of fibers that the manufacturers use in crafting the scope is a trade secret, but it is estimated to range from 10,000 to 20,000 fibers. The sharpness of the fiberoptic view is no better than the actual camera picture.

The scope also has a top-light or direct illumination system. This type of lighting makes viewing slight elevations or depressions difficult, because under direct light they cast no shadows. The intensity of the light also has an important role.

Thirdly, the scope has an extremely wide lens, almost like a fish-eye lens. Therefore, the view is distorted, especially around the edges of the lens.

In addition to these physical limitations of the scope itself, one must also remember that the colon is covered with mucus, which will hinder the view. Peristaltic movements associated with breathing will also disturb the acuity of the view. All these factors contribute to the need to view areas of the colon from a proper distance and under proper light to observe accurately any lesions or abnormalities.

Influenced by the development of the computer technics, endoscopy is about to change. By using some form of computerized endoscopy, the resolution power would increase.

What specific features of the colon make colonoscopic examination difficult?

The mucosa of the colon is attached to the underlying muscle but is not tightly affixed to it. Consequently, the mucosa may droop down and cover the lumen and the haustra, and obstruct the view through the scope. Diverticula associated with narrowing of the lumen also disrupt the view and make finding the true lumen difficult. A dry colon also makes locating the lumen difficult because the mucosa may stick together and thereby close the lumen.

What is the use of taking a photograph through the scope?

Unlike x-ray examinations and other diagnostic tests, a weakness of endoscopic technic is that even though one has means of recording photographically what one sees through the standard scope, endoscopists do not customarily take pictures. This makes intelligent discussion after an examination and evaluation of treatment protocols extremely difficult—and without such discussion, progress will be impossible. Pictures should be taken of lesions and occasionally of the seemingly normal colon for teaching purposes.

Does one make the diagnosis while introducing or withdrawing the colonoscope?

The basis of the endoscopy is "to look before introduction" because once the scope is introduced it is not always possible to distinguish between bleeding due to disease or fresh bleeding from the damage by the scope. To secure the best diagnosis, one should survey the interior of the colon during both introduction and withdrawal. There are advantages and disadvantages to both motions of the scope, as far as viewing the structures within the colon are concerned. The bottom of the haustra is clearly visible in the difficult regions of the colon while the scope is being introduced, but it is sometimes difficult to see the opposite side of the haustra during introduction. The colon looks just like a tube when the scope is being withdrawn, but very often the folds will stick together and make a view of the inside of the haustra difficult if not impossible. You must train yourself to take advantage of every opportunity to view the interior of the colon, whether the scope is being introduced or withdrawn.

Although one may take biopsies with the scope, remember that endoscopy is essentially a visually diagnostic technic. Without experience and ability to

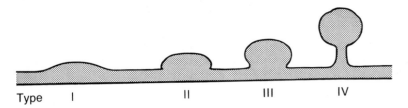

Figure 3–29. Classification of polyps: I, submucosal; II–IV, mucosal.

Type   I   II   III   IV

diagnose a lesion, even selecting the proper place for biopsy is difficult. The endoscopist therefore must develop a "diagnostic eye."

How can one recognize different types of polyps?

Typical cases can be differentiated by recognizing ulcerations, irregularity, size differences, and different consistency or discolorations of tissue, but such observations are not always reliable. It is not difficult to assess whether a polyp is mucosal or submucosal in origin, but this evaluation is often neglected. Yamada and Fukutomi classified stomach polyps in a very simple structural fashion that correlates with malignancy. While this relationship may not apply to the colon, the observation of certain structural features enables the distinction between submucosal and mucosal growths (Fig. 3–29).

When observing a polyp, look for a sharp edge at the base of the polyp. The sharp edge (Fig. 3–29) characterizes a polyp that originates in the mucosa. If the base of the polyp is smooth and gently sloping, or exhibits mucosal bridging, it is a submucosal polyp.

What portion of lesion is biopsied?

The biopsy specimen must come from the exact site where the cancer is suspected. This is why developing skill in diagnosing lesions is essential.

When you biopsy a large ulcer, the specimens should be obtained from the border of the ulcer, not from the crater or the base. When you biopsy a small lesion, the first biopsy specimen is the most important and should be taken from the most suspicious-looking place. It may not be possible to take a second sample because blood may stain the tissues and obscure the lesion. Taking the biopsy from the lowest gravitational point on the tissue will help allay this problem, because any blood that flows from the excision will not obscure the rest of the tissue.

What is the relationship between endoscopy and radiology?

Unfortunately, the endoscopist and the radiologist often view each other as opponents. To secure the best possible information to diagnose a case, both modes of examination should be used to acquire the best possible evaluation of a patient's condition. If an endoscopist feels uncertain about a diagnosis, the radiologist's opinion should be sought. If the radiologist feels uncertain, he should ask the endoscopist to do a biopsy. A good relationship between the two practitioners will ensure the best possible diagnosis.

ENDOSCOPY FOR EVERYBODY

Every doctor can perform endoscopy as long as the proper training and proper skills and knowledge of diagnosis and the technique have been developed. Consequently, more training facilities are needed in order to educate not only the gastroenterologist and colorectal surgeon but also the surgeon and internist. Endoscopy should be performed more frequently because it is a safe, excellent form of examination; but the general principles discussed in this chapter should be observed: do not cause any complications and do not cause the patient any discomfort. If you are uncertain of the diagnosis, send the patient to a specialist in the field. I hope that eventually colonoscopy will help change the statistics of colon cancer and ultimately save lives.

REFERENCES

Cotton, P. B., and Williams, C. B., Practical Gastrointestinal Endoscopy. Blackwell Scientific Publications, Boston, 1980.

Dean, A. C. B., and Shearman, D. J. C., Clinical evaluation of new fiberoptic colonoscope. Lancet, 1:550–552, 1970.

Deyhle, P., Seuberth, K., Jenny, S., and Demling, L., Endoscopic polypectomy in the proximal colon. Endoscopy, 3:103–105, 1971.

Fox, J. A., A fiberoptic colonoscope. Br. Med. J., 3:50, 1969.

Hunt, R. H., and Waye, J. D., Colonoscopy. Chapman and Hall Ltd., 1981.

Hiratsuka, H., How to introduce the colonoscope by rope way method. Gastroenterol. Endosc., 12:209–211, 1970.

Kanazawa, T., Tanaka, Y., and Matsunaga, F., Colonoscopy. Gastroenterol. Endosc., 7:398–400, 1965.

Lemire, S., and Cocco, A. E., Visualization of the left colon with the fiber optic gastroduodenoscope. Gastrointest. Endosc., 13:29–30, 1966.

Makiiski, H., Kitani, A., Kobayashi, K., and Yamamoto, Y., New technique to introduce the colonoscope using the sliding tube. Presented at the 9th annual Autumn Congress of the Japanese Endoscopy Society, September, 1971.

Makiishi, H., Kitano, A., Kobayashi, K., and Yamamoto, Y., A "sliding tube" method available for colonoscopy. Gastroenterol. Endosc., 14:19–101, 1972.

Matsunaga, F., Tajima, T., Toda, S., et al., Colonoscopy. Sogorynsho., 19:325–337, 1970.

Matsunaga, F., Tajima, T., Uno, C., Fiberoscopy and biopsy of the colonic lesions. Clin. Surg., 24:61–357, 1969.

Nagasako, K., Differential Diagnosis of Colorectal Diseases. Igaku-Shoin Ltd., Tokyo, 1982.

Nagasako, K., Nakamura, K., Suzuki, S., et al., Colonoscopy: observation of the ileocecal valve. Gastroenterol. Endosc., 12:212–214, 1970.

Niwa, H., Colonoscopy. Gastroenterol. Endosc., 7:402–408, 1965.

Niwa, H., Complications of colonoscopy. Gastroenterol. Endosc., 21:178–192, 1979.

Niwa, H., Utsumi, Y., Kaneko, E., et al., Colonoscopy. Gastroenterol. Endosc. 11:163–173, 1969.

Oshiba, S., and Watanabe, A., Colonoscopy. Gastroenterol. Endosc., 7:400–402, 1965.

Overhold, B. F., and Pollard, H. M., Cancer of the colon and rectum: current procedures for detection and diagnosis. Cancer, 20:445–450, 1967.

Provenzale, L., Camerada, P., and Revignas, A., La coloscopia totale tranceanale mediante una metodica originale. Rass. Med. Sarda. 69:149–160, 1966.

Rogers, B. H. G., Silvis, S. E., Nebel, O. T., et al., Complications of flexible fiberoptic colonoscopy and polypectomy. Gastroenterol. Endosc., 22:73–77, 1975.

Sakai, Y., Basic knowledge of colonoscopy. Naika., 35:829, 1975.

Sakai, Y., Practical Fiberoptic Colonoscopy. Igaku-Shoin Ltd., Tokyo 1981.

Sakai, Y., Eto, K., Miyaoka, M., et al., Abnormal loop encountered in colonoscopy. Gastroenterol. Endosc., 17:573–580, 1975.

Sakita, T., ed., Gastroendoscopy. (English edition) International Medical Foundation of Japan, 1972.

Schindler, R., Gastroscopy, 2nd ed. Hafner Publishing Co., New York, 1966.

Shinya, H., Colonoscopy. Igaku-Shoin Ltd., Tokyo, 1982.

Shinya, H., Personal communication, 1978.

Sugawa, C., and Schuman, B. M., Primer of Gastrointestinal Fiberoptic Endoscopy. Little, Brown, Co., Boston, 1981.

Torsole, A., Arullani, P., and Casale, C., An application of transintestinal intubation to the study of the colon. Gut, 8:192–194, 1967.

Tsuneoka, K., and Uchida, T., Fibergastroscopic polypectomy with snare method and its significance developed in our department—polyp resection and recovery instruments. Gastroenterol. Endosc., 11:174–184, 1969.

Turell, R., Fiberoptic colonoscope and sigmoidoscope. Am. J. Surg., 105:133–136, 1963.

Yamada, T., and Fukutomi, H., Gastric polyp. Gastroenterol. Endosc., 7:448–450, 1965.

4 CHAPTER

ANESTHESIA

INTRODUCTION

I was trained during my residency years to administer caudal and transacral anesthesia as the routes of choice for anorectal surgery except in pediatric surgery, pelvic abscesses, and certain other conditions which required general anesthesia. Local anesthesia was occasionally used for some in-office surgery.

I adopted these principles early in my practice, but the disadvantages of the various methods were noted over a period of a few years. The caudal block was only effective in about 80 per cent of patients. The transacral block was time-consuming, and anesthesiologists were not always available to administer it. Spinal anesthesia was often feared by the patient and was responsible in some instances for headaches, mild transient neurologic symptoms, and backache. Despite its undesirable side effects, some patients practically demanded general anesthesia for routine anorectal surgery. Intubation was used so that the inverted position could still be employed.

In retrospect, what is surprising is that all types of external surgery in the office, such as for abscesses, pilonidal cysts, and external tags of hemorrhoids, were being performed without knowing how to relax the sphincter mechanism properly.

LOCAL ANESTHESIA

Local anesthesia is really not new, but the technic and agents that produce anesthesia, hemostasis, and relaxation of the anorectal muscles without edema and distortion of the tissue evolved from Schneider, who was the first to add hyaluronidase to the anesthetic agent several decades ago. In 1956, my first resident and I decided that further research was necessary because not all patients responded well, some developing a transient hypertension from the anesthetic agent and requiring vasodilators such as amyl nitrite. All operations by the Allentown Hospital surgeons using local agents for anorectal procedures were carefully monitored by the members of the anesthesiology department. It was difficult to draw conclusions because the four surgeons varied in their technic and the amount of agent injected.

However, the conclusion was that two ampules of hyaluronidase added to the anesthetic agent produced better results than when only one or more than three were added.

In retrospect, it was the anesthetic and not the hyaluronidase that produced the good results. Fortunately, lidocaine became available at approximately the time the research was completed, and all the problems associated with previous local anesthetic agents disappeared. Since then I have used lidocaine in many thousands of patients. Its use is becoming increasingly popular among colorectal specialists in the United States.

Technic

Generally, with anesthesia, the least amount used to achieve the desired result the better. The less interference with normal physiology the better. While in my entire experience I have yet to see a death from local anesthesia, I have seen respiratory depression and drop in blood pressure from too much preoperative sedation given prior to local anesthesia in the hospital. In office practice, to avoid side effects, including nausea, absolutely no preoperative medication is given. There are some tense patients, usually children, who will initially show anxiety and even nausea. Reassurance and a short wait is all that is usually necessary. Very rarely is it necessary to change the patient from the inverted jack-knife to the flat supine position for a few minutes.

The anesthesia must be given as painlessly as possible. If indicated by the medical history, a skin test for allergy may be done, although true allergy to the "-caines" is rare. Using a small hypodermic needle, the initial skin-anesthetizing wheal is raised in the midline one or two inches posterior to the anus. After the wheal is made, the needle is inserted in the subcutaneous tissue and a thin layer of the anesthetic agent is placed covering the entire perianal area, preferably up to the dentate line (Fig. 4–1). Two other injections

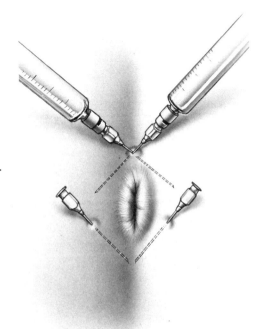

Figure 4–1. Preferred sites for subcutaneous injection of anesthetic agent.

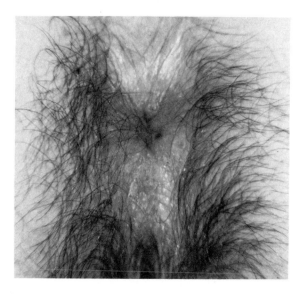

Figure 4–2. Anus before anesthesia.

are made in the already anesthetized skin, thus sparing the patient additional pain. Then gently but firmly the anal area is pressed or "massaged" with a gauze sponge. Frequently one will actually see the anus relax (Figs. 4–2 and 4–3). As in all injections, it is well to aspirate or pull back on the plunger occasionally, although it is rare that the needle will enter a vessel. When blood appears in the syringe all that is necessary is to change the direction of the needle and proceed.

After the subcutaneous area is completely infiltrated, or even before infiltration in obese individuals, the needle is changed to a 2½-inch 24-gauge needle. If there is no sign of anal relaxation, one need not hesitate to inject 1 ml or more of the agent into the external muscle in each of the four quadrants. A finger inserted into the anal canal will determine what size Hill-Ferguson retractor to use to continue the submucosal part of the injection (Fig. 4–4). If a fissure or other painful lesion is present, it is important to anesthetize the base of the fissure even before performing digital examination (Fig. 4–5). If the anal canal is contracted from stricture or scar, the local anesthesia must be completed by working through a small retractor, or, since the skin is

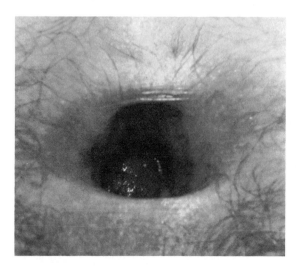

Figure 4–3. Relaxation achieved after anesthesia.

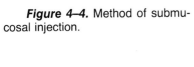
Figure 4–4. Method of submucosal injection.

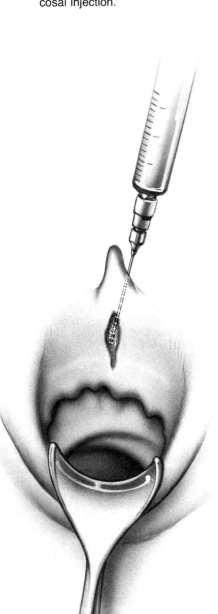

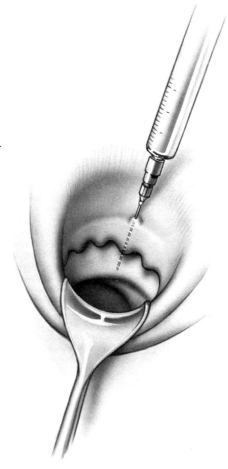

Figure 4–5. Injection at the base of a fissure.

already anesthetized, the scar of fibrous band must be released before instrumentation is introduced. A normal anal canal should accommodate a No. 3 retractor. In actual practice I find it possible to proceed immediately to the No. 3 retractor and use a longer needle, inserting it through the anesthetized skin just distal to the dentate line and onto the submucosal area of the lower rectum. It is important to instill a thin layer of anesthetic agent submucosally in the entire circumference of the anal canal. A common mistake in administering an anesthetic is to inject the agent solely underneath the hemorrhoids or other disease process. However, meticulous work requires complete anesthesia and relaxation of the anorectum. The secret of local anesthesia is that it blocks all the nerves, including those controlling the involuntary mechanisms.

With the exception of a painful fissure, which requires the injection of the anesthetic agent underneath its base early in the anesthetizing process, it is preferable to complete the injections elsewhere prior to injecting potentially infected areas. An anal fistula is one such infected area. Generally the surgeon knows the location of the tract from the patient's history, palpation, or visualization. Figure 4–6 depicts a rectorectal fistula with a tract running in the submucosal tissue from a crypt at the anorectal line to an area several inches higher in the rectum. The anesthetic agent is injected into or just beneath the mucosa around and slightly above the tract, without actually entering the infected area. Occasionally but not often, the agent is injected into the fistulous tract and will be seen at once as it exudes from one of its orifices. The purpose of the anesthetic is not only anesthesia but relaxation and hemostasis, which greatly facilitates the surgery, particularly when placing continuous or interrupted sutures to maintain marsupialization and to ensure hemostasis.

The foregoing procedure produces complete anorectal anesthesia. By no means would one do this for conditions such as external thrombotic hemorrhoids or external abscesses which do not require relaxation of the sphincter mechanism.

For the beginning surgeon I would suggest that pain can be avoided by giving the injections carefully and slowly, and preferably in a hospital, where adequate preoperative or intraoperative sedation is feasible if necessary.

A word about needles: The fine caliber needle is good for subcutaneous injection but a slightly heavier needle should be used for submucosal injection to achieve better manipulation and to avoid the possibility of breakage. This problem is very rare, but it exemplifies the precaution and skill needed to achieve superior results. The art of surgery requires the same care for the most simple procedures as for the most sophisticated operations. There should be no exceptions.

The anesthetic solution consists of lidocaine hydrochloride, 0.5 per cent solution with epinephrine 1:200,000; usually 20 to 35 ml is sufficient. The solution comes already prepared. One ampule of hyaluronidase, a mucolytic enzyme that breaks down tissue barriers and produces a quick, even spread of the anesthetic, is added to the solution just before administration. I use hyaluronidase in hospital practice but seldom in office practice except to quickly reduce the edema of acute hemorrhoidal disease. However, the beginning surgeon should use it, because the use of hyaluronidase will certainly aid in securing a more profound anesthesia.

Figure 4–7 depicts the tray used for local anesthesia.

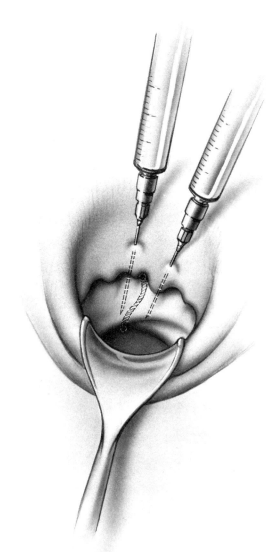

Figure 4–6. Method of injection around a fistula.

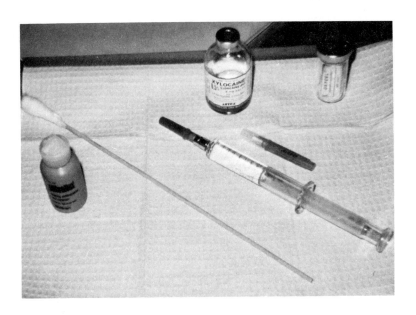

Figure 4–7. Tray for local anesthesia.

Contraindications

Contraindications to local anesthesia include operations in children who cannot cooperate, deep abscess in the retrorectal or pelvic area, extensive fistulous tracts with multiple secondary openings, and sinus tracts such as hidradenitis suppurativa. In other words, local anesthesia is contraindicated where infection is a problem, where more than 100 ml of the anesthetic agent must be used, or where the surgeon doubts that the agent can be safely injected around the areas of infection. The absolute contraindications to local anesthesia are nonlocalized or extensive infection and allergy to the "-caines." When these few exceptions occur, the surgeon is advised to let the anesthesiologist make the necessary decisions.

REFERENCES

Kratzer, G. L., Out-patient anorectal surgery. American Family Physician. March, 1975.

Salvati, E. P., and Kratzer, G. L., Advantages of local over spinal anesthesia in anorectal surgery. Surg. Gynecol. Obstet., *103*:434, 1956.

Schneider, H. C., Personal communication.

CHAPTER 5

ABSCESSES

INTRODUCTION

The management of infection of the anorectal area has three basic characteristics: correct diagnosis, adequate drainage, and the proper use of antibiotics. There are two aspects of the management of anorectal infections that are different from treatment of infection in other parts of the body. These are the greater danger of disturbance of function and the extremely rare indications for antibiotic coverage.

Proper treatment requires a knowledge of the regional anatomy and physiology and of the pathogenesis of anorectal infection. It is easy for the experienced proctologist and difficult for the resident. The inexperienced clinician tends to be too aggressive in the treatment of abscesses and is inclined to literally remove the abscess wall while attempting to perform simultaneous fistulectomy, even in the presence of inflamed and highly friable tissues. When the fistula is simple and has an obvious primary opening, experienced surgeons are more likely to perform only incision and drainage of the abscess and occasionally fistulotomy.

Not all abscesses result in fistulas, or at least not in obvious ones. An overzealous search for a fistula can result in creation of a false passage. The prime objective of treatment is to drain the abscess, which can usually be accomplished in the office, and to search for a possible fistula after all inflammation has subsided. The subsequent fistulotomy can usually be performed in the office. The patient should seldom lose time from work as a result of anorectal abscess. The routine is simple, logical, economical, and safe, and it is less likely to disturb the function of the sphincter mechanism and result in postoperative incontinence and seepage—sequelae of poor or mediocre surgery for anorectal disease.

CLASSIFICATION

Abscesses Not Due to Crypt Infection

In approaching the problem of anorectal infection, the physician should have an open mind and be prepared to adapt the management of the problem

Table 5–1. CLASSIFICATION OF ANORECTAL INFECTIONS

Those Not Due to Crypt Infection*
  Skin infections
  Trauma
  Foreign bodies—ingested or extraneous
  Inflammatory bowel disease
  Septicemia
  Blood dyscrasias

Those Due to Crypt Infection†
Infralevator
  Subcutaneous
  Submucosal
  Intersphincteric
  Superficial postanal
  Deep postanal
  Ischiorectal‡
Supralevator (Deep)
  Pelvirectal
  Retrorectal
  Rectovesical
Unusual
  Primarily involves the abdomen and pelvis

*May be infralevator or supralevator infections.
†The words superficial, deep, and unusual are used arbitrarily mainly in diagnosis. The only pertinent word is "deep." The deep abscess is one that extends above the level of the levator muscle and may involve the supralevator space.
‡May be horseshoe-shaped.

to the patient's situation. Always think of the patient first and the infection second.

There are two types of anorectal infections (Table 5–1). The first does not initially involve the anal canal but may originate from a skin infection around the anal area such as infected hair follicles or furuncles, hidradenitis suppurativa from infected apocrine sweat glands, sinuses from a poorly healing episiotomy wound, Bartholin cyst, or pilonidal disease. I have seen pilonidal sinuses on the perineum and scrotum that had their origin in the sacrococcygeal region, but whose secondary openings occurred at quite distant places. Sinuses in the perianal area can be due to diverticulitis of the sigmoid colon with abscess and fistulization to the perineum without involving the anal canal. Appendicitis, inflammatory bowel disease, periurethral infection, and some presacral tumors can infrequently produce such fistulas or sinuses.

Abscesses in the anorectal area may also be produced by trauma. Injury may be self-inflicted or it may result from accidents or from instrumentation used in diagnostic procedures such as barium enemas. Even vigorous removal of fecal impactions may cause trauma and subsequent abscess. Inflammatory bowel disease, tuberculosis, various blood dyscrasias, particuarly leukemias, and poor resistance from systemic infection such as septicemia may also result in abscesses.

Abscesses Due to Crypt Infection

The second cause of anorectal abscess is infection in the anal crypts and the microscopic anal ducts or glands that have their openings in the anal crypts. These anal glands or ducts penetrate the lower border of the internal sphincter muscle and actually determine the initial route that any given infection will take (Fig. 5–1). Anorectal abscesses can be classified by the

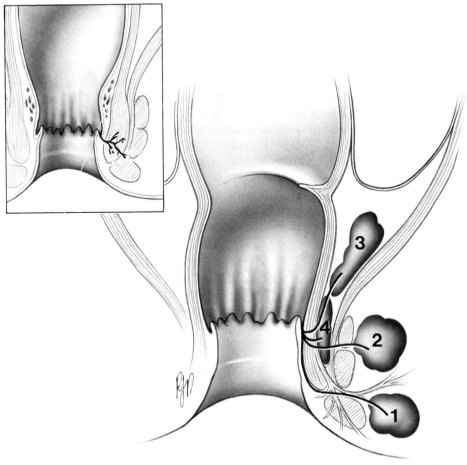

Figure 5–1. Composite picture showing sites of abscesses.

1, Superficial postanal space.
2, Ischiorectal fossa.
3, Supralevator space.
4, Intersphincteric space.
   Inset, Diagram showing the anal ducts penetrating the internal sphincter and the various directions in which infection can spread.

anatomic location where they occur (Table 5–1). When first seen, the infection and the abscess it creates may be limited to the subcutaneous or submucosal area, as in abscesses associated with fissure. The infection may be limited to the area around the subcutaneous external sphincter muscle or to the intersphincteric area. The latter abscess is situated between the internal and external sphincter, and may be either low or high in reference to the dentate line. An abscess may be limited to the ischiorectal area or it may be limited to the deep postanal space. These anatomic spaces, termed *infralevator,* constitute the common areas in which abscesses occur. Anorectal abscesses would be relatively easy to diagnose and treat if they all remained limited to these spaces. Unfortunately, because of either the virulence of the infection, the unnecessary use of antibiotics, or delay on the part of the patient or physician, these infectious processes often spread quickly to other areas and involve multiple spaces. An abscess in the deep postanal space may easily extend laterally on one or both sides to the ischiorectal fossae. If both these fossae are involved, the abscess is known as a posterior horseshoe-shaped abscess. The intermuscular abscess may extend anteriorly to the deep anterior rectal space, which is between the superficial and deep external sphincter muscles, and subsequently involve the ischiorectal fossae. When this happens, it is known as an anterior horseshoe-shaped abscess. Such abscesses may involve the rectovaginal septum and, although rare, can cause a rectovaginal fistula.

Ischiorectal abscesses occasionally break through the levator muscle to involve the *supralevator* space (Fig. 5–2). Intersphincteric abscesses may extend cephalad to become high intersphincteric abscesses and sometimes they involve the supralevator space by breaking through the conjoined longitudinal muscle of the rectum into the pelvirectal, retrorectal, or rectovesical spaces.

At the risk of sounding too simplistic, understanding the anatomy and infectious processes at the anorectal area becomes easier if we think of the anal canal in terms of layers of tissue and circles. Keep in mind that for the most part when we refer to spaces where abscesses may occur, there is always the potential for such infection to completely encircle the anorectal area in that particular plane. Extensive infection can cut across planes, and, for that matter, extremely virulent infection, especially that caused by the anaerobic organisms, may extend quickly and break through any fascial planes to

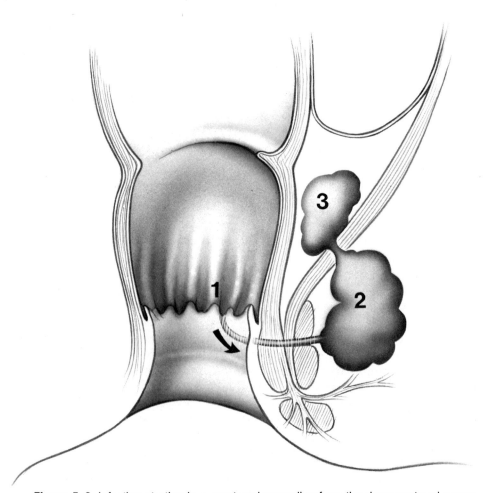

Figure 5–2. Infection starting in a crypt and spreading from the deep postanal space *(1)* to the ischiorectal fossa *(2)*, and then extending to supralevator space *(3)*.

involve all perirectal, pelvic, scrotal, thigh, or vulvar tissues. Fortunately, the great majority of abscesses and fistulas are superficial and relatively simple to treat.

The first plane, then, starting within the lumen of the surgical anal canal and working outward, is the *subcutaneous* or *submucosal* space. As is true of all planes of the anorectal area, infection may involve any portion or the entire circumference of this space to be described.

Between the internal and external sphincter muscles is the second plane or space, called the *intersphincteric space*. Intersphincteric abscesses may be described as high or low, depending on whether they extend above or below the dentate line.

The external sphincter muscle comprises three parts. The first part, known as the subcutaneous portion, is circular and relatively small. The small or superficial postanal abscess occurs most frequently posterior and adjacent to the subcutaneous portion of the external sphincter. It may occur anywhere in this perisubcutaneous external sphincter plane.

The second and largest portion of the external sphincter muscle is known as the superficial portion. It decussates anteriorly and posteriorly and is attached to the tip of the coccyx and perineum, respectively. The area around this muscle is known as the perisuperficial external sphincter plane.

The deep portion of the external sphincter is circular and blends with the inferior border of puborectalis. The deep postanal abscess occurs adjacent to the muscle, and as the name accurately implies, it frequently occurs posteriorly. The area around this muscle forms still another circular plane. It communicates with the ischiorectal fossae and when infected may form horseshoe-shaped fistulae.

The third and highest circular plane of the rectum is the *supralevator space*. It is not a true anatomic circle because this space is divided between the retrorectal and pelvirectal areas by fascial attachments.

It should be emphasized that these planes have been described merely to simplify the normal anatomy and make infectious processes more understandable. Both the normal tissues and the extent of infection are palpable. Always remember that infection can spread slowly or rapidly in any direction, depending on the virulence of the invading organism and the resistance of the host.

Classification of abscesses and fistulas is a recent and extremely helpful innovation. Parks of England deserves much of the credit, although the basis for classification originated from Chiari's description of the anal glands.

Anal crypts and anal ducts or glands are more numerous in the posterior portion of the anal canal, and abscesses are also more frequent in that region. Extensive abscesses creating curved or angulated fistulas are more apt to originate in a crypt posteriorly because of the greater prevalence of anal ducts in this area. Abscesses of all varieties occurring in the anterior portion of the anal canal are apt to form straight, easily healed fistulas because there are fewer ducts in this area. Abscesses occur least frequently in the lateral portions of the canal, where ducts and crypts are sparse.

Infection begins in a crypt and burrows into the anal ducts. An abscess may form in the subcutaneous or submucosal areas and the infection may stop there or drain back through the crypt of origin, thus forming a "blind" fistula. Unless surgically drained, it may also open spontaneously. Infection may continue through all or a portion of the subcutaneous external sphincter muscle and an abscess may form at the anal verge, or it may take a deeper course into the deep postanal space, forming an abscess superior to the anococcygeal raphe and posterior to the deep bundle of the external sphincter muscle. If not surgically drained, it may break into either or both ischiorectal fossae and may become horseshoe shaped. The infection may follow the fascial planes in almost any direction, breaking through Colles' fascia to the scrotum or through the levator muscle or fascia to involve the supralevator spaces, and even extending through the conjoined longitudinal coat of the rectum, leaving a fistula. If the patient survives the extensive infection, this kind of anorectal abscess is difficult to cure without causing complete fecal incontinence. Fortunately, these abscesses frequently rupture spontaneously through the skin overlying the ischiorectal fossae before pursuing a more catastrophic course (Fig. 5–3).

Still another pathway for infection from the crypt is along the anal glands, ultimately penetrating the lower portion of the internal sphincter muscle and forming a low or high intersphincteric abscess. If not drained intra-anally or intrarectally, the infection may break through the mucosa of the rectum, leaving a rectorectal fistula, which is not difficult to treat. Or it may extend and end in a blind pouch in the supralevator area or cause an

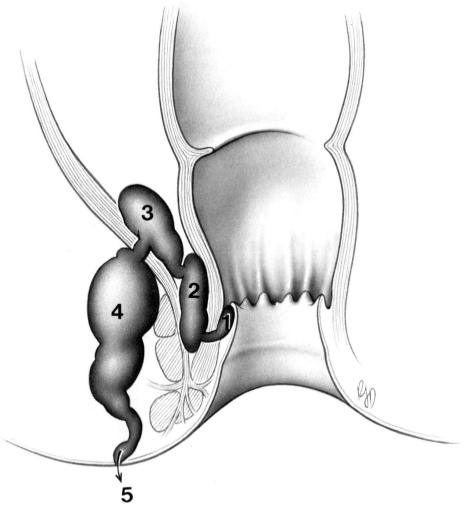

Figure 5–3. Neglected abscess may begin in a crypt *(1)*, extend to the intersphincteric area *(2)*, break through into the supralevator space *(3)*, extend to the ischiorectal fossa *(4)*, and then form a secondary opening on the skin of the perianal region *(5)*.

abscess in the supralevator space, which is still not too difficult to treat if it is recognized early.

DIAGNOSIS

HISTORY

Since many of my patients are under the care of an internist or primary care physician, a history and physical examination have already been performed. However, it is advisable for a member of the office staff to inquire about family history, past medical history, social history, and allergies. Past and present medications and information about bleeding tendencies are also important. I prefer to question the patient myself concerning the history of the present illness and special symptoms relating to the gastrointestinal tract and particularly the rectum. This includes questions about bleeding, itching, anal protrusion, abdominal or rectal pain, diarrhea, and constipation (Table 5–2). This information is helpful in differentiating the type of abscess present. The patient with possible anorectal abscess is almost certain to have pain because practically all anorectal abscesses start in the anal canal and extend outward toward the skin. The pain usually has been present for several days before the patient comes to the office. It is persistent, constant, and throbbing in nature, and becomes progressively worse. The patient can usually tell the doctor exactly where the pain is and may also offer the information that there is swelling or firmness in the painful area, which may be anywhere in the perianal region. The vast majority of anorectal abscesses do not produce general symptoms such as fever and chills, but it is advisable to inquire about these other symptoms. Fever and chills with a feeling of heaviness in the rectal area indicate the presence of a rather deep ischiorectal abscess or a deep, virulent infection, which should alert one to proceed with caution.

Abscesses may be caused by many organisms including those that make up the normal intestinal flora. It is therefore necessary to do routine cultures and sensitivity tests on the exudate. Both aerobic and anaerobic organisms must be considered. Very rarely the tubercle bacillus, parasites, and fungi such as *Actinomyces* must be considered.

INSPECTION AND DIGITAL EXAMINATION

The perianal area should be inspected. Naturally, a firm, painful, or tender, reddened area is pathognomonic of abscess. However, I find that it is best to explore the anorectal area thoroughly in all cases, and if there is not

Table 5–2. DIAGNOSIS OF ANORECTAL ABSCESS

Symptom	Type of Abscess		
	Superficial	*Deep*	*Unusual*
Pain	Yes	Possible	Possible
Swelling	Yes	No	Possible
Tenderness	Yes	Possible	Possible
Anal spasm	Yes	No	No
Fever	No	Yes	Yes
Systemic reaction	No	Yes	Yes
Sensation of rectal fullness	No	Yes	Possible
Peritoneal irritation	No	No	Yes
Abdominal mass	No	No	Possible
Pelvic mass	No	No	Possible

too much pain, it is important to perform a digital examination, using the right index finger inserted into the anal canal and rectum and the thumb of the same hand on the outside of the anus. In an effort to determine the extent of the abscess and if either subcutaneous or submucosal induration is present at the anorectal line, the index finger can be curved around and above the levator muscle to meet the thumb externally. In this fashion it is possible to determine which quadrants of the anorectal area are indurated and whether there is any pelvic bogginess or evidence of any supralevator extension. Such an extension will not be found often, but it is important to rule out a complicated abscess, which might require that the patient be hospitalized for examination and management. Induration in the anal canal or the perianal area even without fluctuation confirms the diagnosis, and the treatment is simple. Induration beginning at the dentate line and proceeding superiorly and posteriorly, with fluctuation or a sense of fullness or firmness in the deep postanal space, is diagnostic of a deep postanal space abscess. Induration of the deep postanal space and both ischiorectal fossae is indicative of a posterior horseshoe-shaped abscess. Induration superior to the main bulk of the external sphincter mechanism anteriorly, with induration of both ischiorectal fossae, suggests an anterior horseshoe-shaped abscess. Induration that can be palpated approximately at the intersphincteric groove and involving only the rectal wall extending superiorly in the anal canal towards the rectal area with a normal ischiorectal fossae indicates the presence of an intersphincteric abscess. It is important to follow this relatively narrow superior extension in the intermuscular wall of the rectum to see whether the induration tends to go toward the lumen of the rectum or toward the rectal mucosa, or whether it proceeds above the levator muscle into the supralevator space. If such an abscess has broken into the supralevator space, there will be a sense of fullness and bogginess in that part of the supralevator space. If the abscess is an extensive or neglected one, it is possible for pus to extend around the lower rectum in a circular fashion to involve the entire supralevator space.

Another example of an extensive anorectal infection is one characterized by induration and fluctuation of both of the ischiorectal fossae, with induration or bogginess in the supralevator space. This probably means that the patient had a neglected ischiorectal abscess that extended through the levator muscle into the supralevator space to form abscesses in that area. Supralevator or pelvic infection with abscess formation due to causes other than that of anal crypt and anal gland infection have general and abdominal symptoms that establish the diagnosis. I have seen several cases of diverticulitis with abscess formation in the pelvis that caused perforation of the levator fascia or muscle with involvement of the ischiorectal fossa and creation of a sinus to the perianal area. I have also seen diverticulitis patients with fecal fistulae into the vagina. In diagnosing anorectal abscesses, one should be alert for pilonidal abscesses that extend very close to the anus and sometimes circumvent the anus in an anterior fashion and open on the perineum. Bartholin's gland infection can also be confusing, but with careful inspection and digital examination as described, there should be no difficulty in differentiating it. Abscesses from poorly healing episiotomy wounds are usually superficial but occasionally may cause a low rectovaginal fistula. Presacral tumors are not easily confused with retrorectal abscess, but sometimes they present with an abscess in either the retrorectal space or the perianal area. It is difficult to quote the actual incidence of the various types of abscesses, but my experience agrees with that of Goligher, in that superficial and ischiorectal abscesses are more frequently encountered and superlevator abscesses are rare.

INSTRUMENTATION

Examination by anoscopy, proctoscopy, or sigmoidoscopy is of limited value in the diagnosis of the acute anorectal abscess. Such an examination will cause varying amounts of pain. The small-caliber pediatric sigmoidoscope will generally provide the important visual findings within the anal canal, rectum, and lower sigmoid colon. Pus seen exuding from a crypt or an opening in the rectum, and the presence of ulcerative proctosigmoiditis may be helpful in the differential diagnosis and location of an abscess. Pelvic abscess or diverticular disease may limit the length of insertion of the instrument, which may be useful diagnostic information.

TREATMENT

Anorectal infection or abscesses should be considered an emergency situation. Infections spread quickly, and it is very important to drain the area before the abscess enters new tissue space. The vast majority of anorectal abscesses are due to crypt infection, and many of these may be managed as an office procedure, with incision and drainage accomplished using local anesthesia. This is possible because most abscesses in this area tend to point toward the perianal skin surface. However, patients with large abscesses with diffuse cellulitis, those who are obese or large and have long anal canals, or those who show signs of systemic reaction usually require hospitalization, with incision and drainage carried out under spinal or general anesthesia. Pediatric patients usually require general anesthesia, although in some instances local anesthesia in the office may be employed. Abscesses due to trauma, foreign bodies, inflammatory bowel disease, septicemia, and the blood dyscrasias are best treated in the hospital. In addition to wide drainage of the perineum or perineal area, trauma and foreign bodies may require abdominal exploration with colostomy.

It is not possible to anesthetize an abscess, but after an appraisal of the size and type of abscess involved, it is usually easy to anticipate the length of the skin incision required for adequate drainage. The local anesthetic agent can be injected intradermally over the area to be incised (Fig. 5–4). I find it useful to make crisscross incisions and excise a small portion of the skin in order to keep the wound open. Bleeding from the skin is easily controlled with the Hyfrecator. If this is not available, Oxycel gauze may be placed in the abscess cavity not only to keep the wound open, but also to provide satisfactory hemostasis. A pressure dressing using a roll of gauze and adhesive to strap the buttock together will usually prevent annoying oozing. It is important to explain to the patient that anorectal abscesses will leave a residual fistula in approximately 65 per cent of patients.

Abscesses presenting on the perianal skin do not require relaxation of the sphincter mechanism for drainage. However, abscesses occurring in the anal canal and even submucosal abscesses above the dentate line, including intersphincteric abscesses, necessitate relaxation of the sphincter muscle. These can be drained under local anesthesia provided that the local anesthetic agent is first given subcutaneously circumferentially. The anesthetic agent used is not injected in any indurated area until relaxation of the sphincter mechanism occurs to such an extent that a small retractor can be placed in the anal canal and a small amount of anesthetic agent can be given submucosally before the incision and drainage. In this type of abscess, it is important

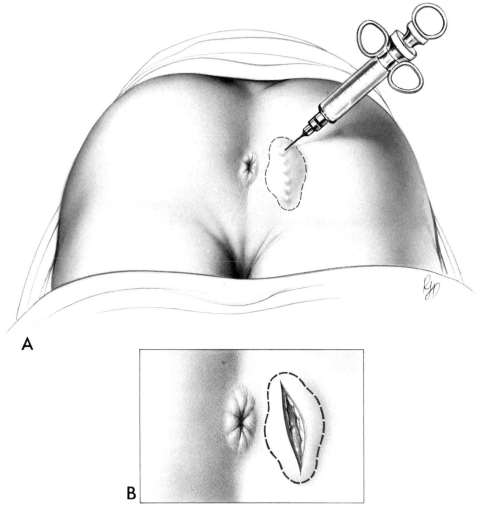

Figure 5–4. *A,* Intradermal injection overlying the ischiorectal abscess. *B,* Extent of incision of skin.

to extend the incision out well beyond the anal verge for drainage and proper healing (Fig. 5–5).

The superficial abscesses present no particular problem for incision and drainage in the office (Fig. 5–6). The occasional operator may question the wisdom of draining a rather deep postanal abscess or deep ischiorectal abscess. If reasonably certain that the abscess is indeed limited to one of these areas, I do not hesitate to anesthetize the skin and subcutaneous tissues and muscle until the abscess cavity is reached (Figs 5–6 and 5–7). I make certain that a wide enough area of the skin and the subcutaneous tissues is included to make adequate drainage possible (Fig. 5–8). However, if there is any question, especially in large, obese patients with long anal canals, the safest and best course to follow is hospitalization, where the appropriate anesthesia may be administered. The supralevator abscesses are extremely rare and certainly require hospitalization and regional or general anesthesia (Fig. 5–9). Very rarely a patient will present with an overwhelming infection resulting in abscesses involving practically all of the perirectal spaces and adjacent structures. These patients require extensive drainage performed under general anesthesia.

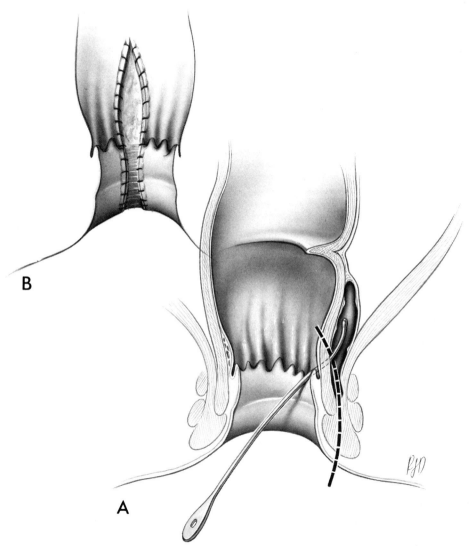

Figure 5–5. *A,* Probe inserted through involved crypt into abscess cavity. Tissue overlying the probe is incised. This incision is extended caudad well beyond the anal verge. Interrupted line indicates the usual incision required. *B,* The wound is completely marsupialized to control bleeding and facilitate healing.

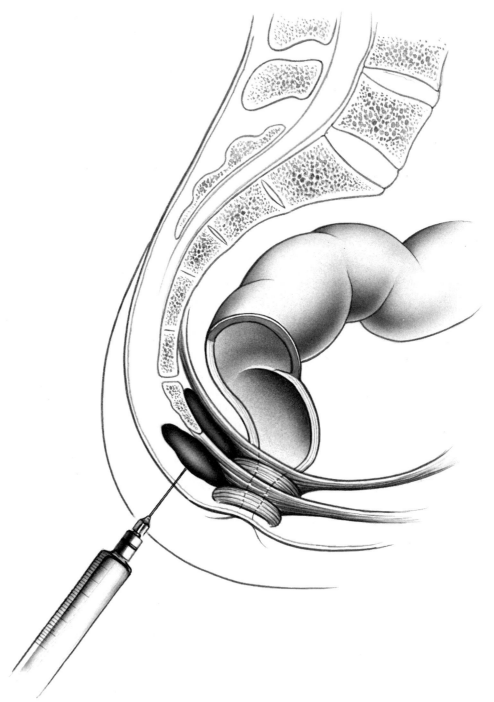

Figure 5–6. Method of injecting anesthetic agent for abscesses in the superficial and deep postanal spaces.

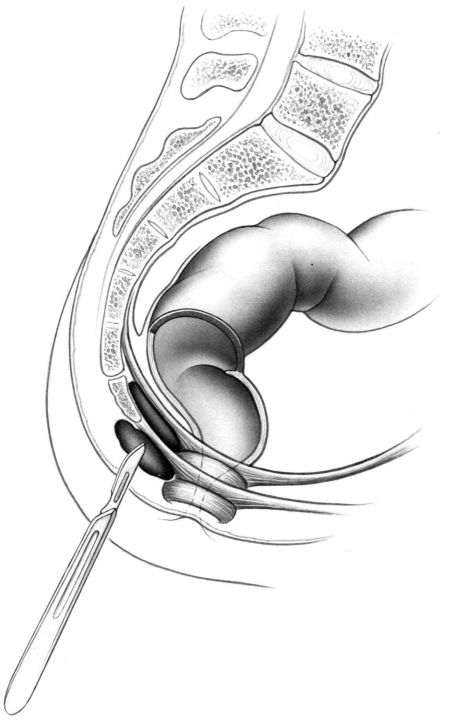

Figure 5–7. Hilton's method sometimes used in deep postanal abscesses after initial incision of skin and subcutaneous tissues.

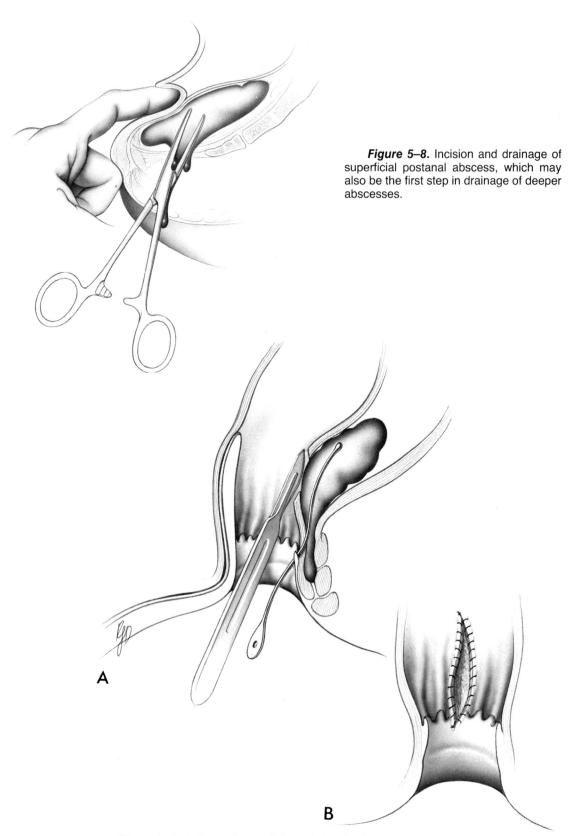

Figure 5–8. Incision and drainage of superficial postanal abscess, which may also be the first step in drainage of deeper abscesses.

A

B

Figure 5–9. *A,* Probe inserted through involved crypt into abscess cavity if possible. Incision and drainage of abscess. *B,* Marsupialization of wound edges.

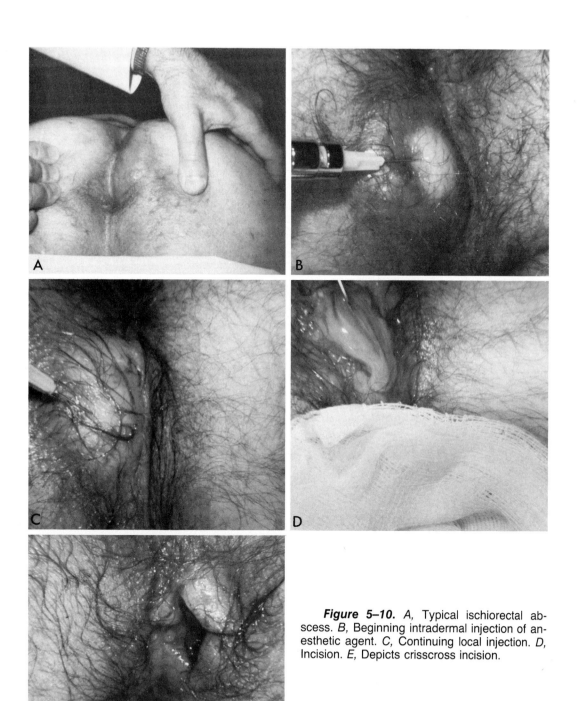

Figure 5–10. *A,* Typical ischiorectal abscess. *B,* Beginning intradermal injection of anesthetic agent. *C,* Continuing local injection. *D,* Incision. *E,* Depicts crisscross incision.

The reader is referred to the discussion of anesthesia in Chapter 4 and to Figure 5–10 *A–E,* which depicts every step in the management of the usual type of abscess.

REFERENCES

Chiari, H., Med. J. Wiess, 419, 1878.
Goligher, J. C., Surgery of the Anus, Rectum, and Colon, 4th ed., Baillière Tindall, London, 1980, p. 156.
Kratzer, G. L., Anal ducts and their clinical significance. Am. J. Surg., 79::34, 1950.
Parks, A. G., Personal communication, 1982.

CHAPTER 6

ANAL FISTULA

INTRODUCTION

A fistula is an abnormal communication between two areas. It is a fibrous tunnel lined by granulation tissue. Anorectal fistulas originate in an anal crypt, where infection begins and extends into the anal glands and through the internal sphincter muscle to form an abscess in either the subcutaneous or the submucosal area. Fistulas may be more extensive when one or more of the pararectal spaces are involved. They are usually preceded by an abscess, but not all abscesses result in fistulas.

Management of most fistulas is routine. Some, however, demand a level of expertise greater than that required for other surgical problems in colon and rectal surgery. A few cannot be cured without risking potential or actual incontinence and other complications.

DIAGNOSIS

It is not possible to overemphasize the value of digital palpation in detecting the induration that indicates the direction of a fistulous tract. Gentle probing is exceedingly important, since the most frequent error in the conduct of fistula surgery is the creation of a false passage. Fistulas that have been present for months or years are easily palpated because of the large amount of fibrous tissue which they contain. It is a mistake to use methylene blue or other staining agents to identify the tract because the fibers and granulation tissue detected by palpation and observation can often provide the landmarks needed for proper fistulectomy.

It is important to emphasize that proper terminology be used to describe the behavior of fistulas. With reference to openings, it is preferable to use the terms primary and secondary rather than internal and external. The primary opening is always internal, usually located in an anal crypt, but the secondary openings are not always external.

There is usually only one primary opening, but there may be several secondary openings. The term "watering pot" is frequently used to describe the condition in which several openings are present on the skin surface. However, these openings communicate with each other and are easy to treat.

Salmon's law (Goodsall's rule) helps locate the primary opening in relation to the secondary (external) opening.[1] If a secondary fistulous opening occurs in the anterior half of the perianal area canal, the primary opening is usually found in the anterior half of the anal canal. Fistulas in this area are usually simple to treat because the tract tends to be straight and short. If a secondary opening occurs in the posterior half of the perianal area, the primary opening is generally located in a crypt of the posterior portion of the anal canal. In fact, the complex fistula generally has its primary opening in the posterior portion of the anal canal. If the fistula has several secondary openings and one is located in the posterior half of the perianal area, the chances are excellent that the primary opening will be found in the posterior half of the anal canal.

Classification. Anorectal fistulas can be classified according to anatomic location, as shown in Table 6–1.

TREATMENT

Local anesthesia can be used for management of practically any anal fistula, provided the anesthetic agent is injected around and not into the fistulous tract (p. 57). The principle behind fistulotomy is simply to convert a pipeline into an open ditch. All that remains is to trim the edges of the overhanging skin to ensure a smooth wound and to secure hemostasis with the Hyfrecator. Fistulotomy is preferred to fistulectomy, excision of the entire tract, because the wound heals quickly and there is less chance of interfering with normal function.

INCOMPLETE OR BLIND FISTULA

The term fistula is occasionally used incorrectly. For instance, an infection may start in a crypt and proceed through the anal glands, form an abscess anywhere in the wall of the anorectum or in the pararectal spaces, and drain spontaneously back through the crypt of origin. This is called a blind fistula (Fig. 6–1A).

The blind fistula is usually relatively superficial. Diagnosis is simply made by using a malleable probe and bending it to form a crypt hook of variable length to conform to the depth of the cavity. A blind fistula can be differentiated from a true or complete fistula because it ends in a blind abscess cavity. This is determined by the fact that at a certain point the probe cannot be advanced further.

Table 6–1. CLASSIFICATION OF FISTULAS

Infralevator
Subcutaneous
Submucosal
Intersphincteric
Postanal
Ischiorectal*

Supralevator
Retrorectal
Pelvirectal
Rectovesical

*May be horseshoe-shaped.

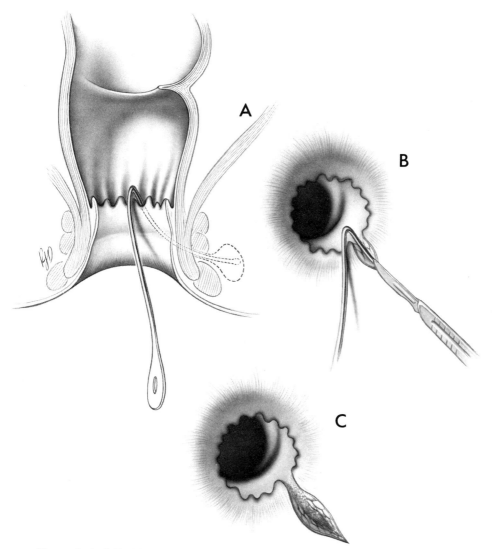

Figure 6–1. *A,* Probing the blind or incomplete fistula. *B,* Boldly cutting over the probe and extending the incision out on the skin for adequate drainage. *C,* The completed incision.

One must cut boldly over the probe to uncap the abscess cavity entirely (Fig. 6–1*B*). If the abscess is superficial, as it usually is, the skin and the superficial portion of the external sphincter muscle must also be cut to drain the cavity to the skin surface. The skin edges should be trimmed to make a smooth wound (Fig. 6–1*C*). A Hyfrecator can be used to control any bleeding. If mucosa must be cut to uncap the cavity thoroughly, a running suture of triple 0 chromic catgut is used to ensure hemostasis and to keep the wound open.

If the blind fistula extends above the dentate line, involves only the mucosa, or appears to run above the sphincter mechanism, marsupialization is all that is necessary. A blind fistula that does not seem to run toward the skin surface does not need drainage or cutting of the muscle or skin. They will heal spontaneously, providing overhanging edges are cut to avoid any kind of pocket, or space for entrapment of infection.

Infralevator Fistula

SUBCUTANEOUS FISTULA

The subcutaneous fistula can usually be palpated as a spoke-like config-uration starting at an anal crypt and extending the length of the anal canal to the anal verge. When pressure is exerted by the finger, a drop of pus will exude from either end of the tract. These fistulas are common and can be easily managed in the office (Fig. 6–2).

The most important step in any fistula surgery is to find the primary opening. The second most important step is to find the secondary opening or openings. The third most important step is to pass a malleable probe through the entire fistulous tract. However, fistulous tracts are not always straight lines but may be angulated or circuitous in nature. If it is not possible to pass a probe throughout the entire course of the fistula, it is important to start with the secondary opening. Letting the probe lead the way, follow the fibrous tract, cutting a little at a time until the primary opening is reached.

Subcutaneous fistulas are not difficult to probe by passing a malleable probe from the secondary opening, through the tract, and out through the primary opening. This, of course, is attempted after the patient has been anesthetized. It is good practice to have the index finger in the anal canal as a guide when one is attempting to pass the probe. After the tip of the probe enters the anal canal, it is easy to bend the tip of the probe and bring it out through the anus. With a Hill-Ferguson retractor in place, all tissues over-lying the probe can be easily incised. Sometimes the primary opening is covered with a thin layer of epithelial tissue. However, if one is sure of the main tract and that a false passage is not being created, one should not hesitate to give the probe an extra push when the suspected crypt is reached.

It is not possible to overemphasize the value of digital palpation in detecting the induration which indicates the direction of a fistulous tract.

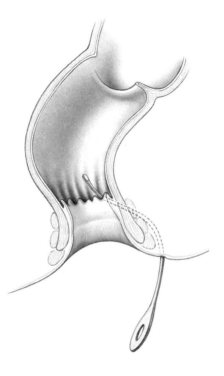

Figure 6–2. Probing the subcutaneous and similar fistulas.

Gentle probing is exceedingly important since the most frequent error in the conduct of fistula surgery is the creation of a false passage.

Fistulas which have been present for months or years are easily palpated because of the large amount of fibrous tissue which they contain. The probe is less apt to produce a "false passage."

SUBMUCOSAL FISTULA

The submucosal fistula produces infection in an anal crypt that extends superiorly under the mucosa and opens onto the rectum between ½ and 3 inches above the dentate line (Fig. 6–3). The probe is passed from the crypt along the fistula and out through the mucosa into the rectum. The overlying tissues are incised and the mucosa trimmed slightly, making it possible for a hemostatic continuous suture of triple 0 chromic catgut so that the submucosal vessels are included. These patients require a few days of bed rest to prevent postoperative bleeding. Many submucosal fistulas, especially those occurring in women, can also be managed in the office.

INTERSPHINCTERIC FISTULA

Management of the intersphincteric fistula is similar to that of the subcutaneous and submucosal fistulas, except that the intersphincteric fistula is deeper and usually involves both the subcutaneous and the submucosal spaces. Since the fistula may penetrate the internal sphincter muscle, it is important to incise the involved portion of the sphincter muscle. It is equally important to extend the incision well beyond the anal verge and to trim any redundant skin, to avoid formation of skin tags and permit proper drainage. The intersphincteric fistula is common, and successful management requires that the patient refrain from physical work for 5 to 10 days following surgery.

POSTANAL SPACE FISTULA

As noted previously, these fistulas are superficial or deep. Superficial postanal space fistula originates in an abscess posterior to the subcutaneous

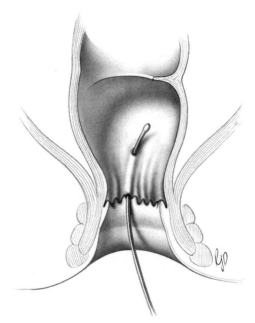

Figure 6–3. Probing the submucosal fistula.

portion of the external sphincter muscle. It is common, readily diagnosed, and easily treated in the same manner as that described for the subcutaneous fistula. The deep postanal space fistula originates in the space posterior to the deep portion of the external sphincter muscle and its management is the same as that for ischiorectal fistula (Fig. 6–4).

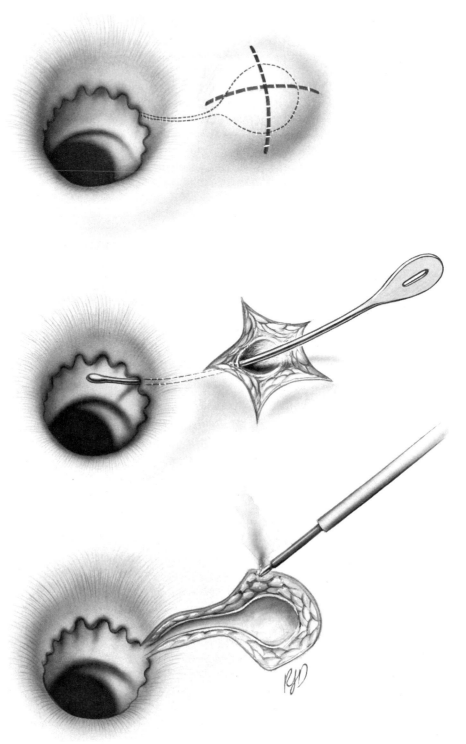

Figure 6–4. Probing and management of the postanal and ischiorectal fistulas.

ISCHIORECTAL AND HORSESHOE-SHAPED FISTULAS

The ischiorectal fistula deserves special attention because it frequently cannot be probed in its entirety before it is incised. Furthermore, this fistula usually occurs in obese, muscular male patients, making its evaluation even more difficult. It is necessary to hospitalize these patients and to use regional anesthesia. These patients usually present with a draining secondary opening over one or both of the ischiorectal fossae. It is possible to palpate the induration of the fistula passing from the secondary opening, through the ischiorectal fossa, and into the deep postanal space. If a horseshoe-shaped fistula is present, induration in the opposite ischiorectal fossa will also be noted. If in doubt regarding the diagnosis, it is better to treat the condition as though a posterior horseshoe-shaped fistula is present.

The primary opening of the fistula is usually found in an anal crypt in the midline posteriorly. It is important to search until the primary opening is identified because, as with all true fistulas, abscesses will continue to occur until the source of infection is removed. With a probe in the primary opening in the midline, it is advisable to insert another probe through the secondary opening to see whether the two probes meet. If they meet, the operative procedure is greatly simplified. If they do not meet, which is usually the case, attempt to pass a probe that has been made into a crypt hook, with a right or slightly acute angle, through the crypt and into the deep postanal space. When this is done, a scalpel should be used to open this space widely and the incision continued externally to cut the fibers of the decussating superficial external sphincter muscle in their longitudinal direction. The subcutaneous external sphincter muscle is then incised, revealing the probe from the secondary opening. The skin and subcutaneous tissue can be cut in the direction of the secondary opening overlying the ischiorectal fossa. The skin and other tissues can be trimmed at this point, depending on the amount of hemorrhoidal tissue present, and a running deep suture of catgut can be used to marsupialize the entire tract. This will ensure hemostasis and keep the wound open for proper drainage.

When treating a posterior horseshoe-shaped fistula, it is important not to continue the incision in the skin and subcutaneous tissue to the other limb of the fistula or secondary opening, should one be present. All that is necessary is to incise the skin and subcutaneous tissue over the opposite ischiorectal space down to the indurated area of that particular limb of the horseshoe-shaped fistula. Since the primary opening has been incised, the cause of the fistula has been removed and the secondary tracts will heal spontaneously whether or not they are curetted. Horseshoe-shaped fistulas can also occur anteriorly, and management is similar to that described for those situated posteriorly.

After inspection for hemostasis, Oxycel gauze is placed in the wound and external pressure is applied. Marsupialization of deep fistulas allows good healing and avoids the necessity for digital examination and other painful procedures in the postoperative period. It is only necessary to see that the skin edges of the wound remain separated. The patient should take sitz baths and must avoid straining at bowel movement for the first 12 days. I see no objection to the use of mineral oil or milk of magnesia in appropriate doses. A high-residue, well-balanced diet is indicated for these patients following surgery.

Figures 6–5 to 6–8 show the essential steps in management of a typical infralevator fistula.

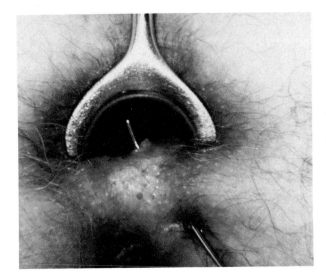

Figure 6–5. Probe in fistulous tract.

Figure 6–6. Tract completely incised.

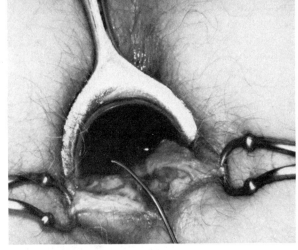

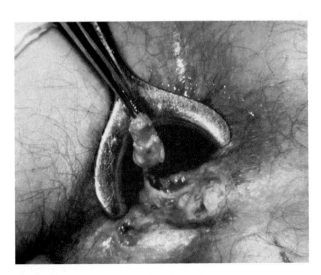

Figure 6–7. Trimming excess skin.

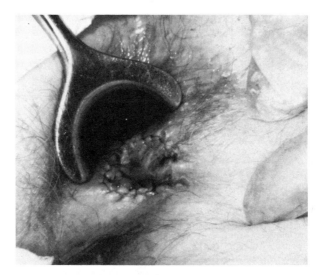

Figure 6–8. Marsupialization completes the operation.

Supralevator Fistulas

Fortunately, supralevator fistulas are quite rare. They can be classified as retrorectal, pelvirectal, and rectovesical. These fistulas demand special diagnostic skills. The examiner must first decide whether the supralevator space(s) are really involved or whether a large ischiorectal abscess that is bulging up against the levator muscle is being palpated. If a supralevator space is involved, it is crucial to determine if this is due to pelvic or abdominal disease or if it is due to an infection originating in the anal crypts, extending superiorly in the intersphincteric space, and breaking through the longitudinal wall of the rectum into the supralevator space. If the ischiorectal fossa is free of induration, but the induration extends from a crypt superiorly above the levator muscle and towards one of the supralevator spaces, this may indicate a blind fistula that originates in a crypt and extends only into the supralevator space. It is important to know the patient's medical history, especially regarding any previous anorectal abscesses and their treatment. If an abscess was opened intrarectally, it means that the crypt of origin was not removed at surgery, which suggests that a probe passed through the primary opening or the involved crypt superiorly either would proceed to a blind end in one of the supralevator spaces or would continue superiorly and lead to a secondary opening in the rectal lumen. The tissues can then be incised over the probe and hemostasis obtained by proper marsupialization of the wound edges.

Again, proper diagnosis of these fistulas is crucial. A secondary opening higher in the rectum certainly indicates that the patient could have had a supralevator abscess that ruptured into the rectum. However, if a secondary opening is not found, one must be quite certain by careful palpation of the ischiorectal fossa of the involved side that the patient does not have a fistula that extends from a crypt superiorly into the supralevator area and then downward into the ischiorectal area and out to the skin surface (a suprasphincteric fistula, in Parks' classification). Along with the findings on palpation, a secondary opening in the skin makes the diagnosis easier. Management of the suprasphincteric fistula is extremely difficult, because the conventional treatment that involves opening the tract would require incision of the entire anorectal ring, which could result in incontinence.

To preserve continence, these patients require a completely diverting colostomy followed by drainage of the involved ischiorectal fossa and closure of the fistula intrarectally. However, an extensive procedure such as this is more likely to be required with the extrasphincteric fistula, which has a direct opening from the perineal skin to the rectum high above the anorectal ring, and not the suprasphincteric fistula, which is due to crypt infection. In many cases of the latter, the use of a modification of the lay-open method may still be possible.

POSTOPERATIVE CARE

Providing wounds have been constructed properly to facilitate drainage and avoid skin tags, the care of the patient following operations for fistula is surprisingly simple. Since the majority of fistula wounds will have an opening on the perianal skin, it is important to avoid "bridging," or premature closing of the skin edges. This can be avoided by gently separating the skin edges of the wound on the second day following the operation. Digital examination is not usually performed until the patient returns to the office on the twelfth postoperative day. At this time the contour of the entire wound can be verified with a well-lubricated finger. This keeps the wound open. By the twelfth day, the patient should have discontinued the use of mineral oil or other laxatives and should have regained control of formed stools.

The surgeon who has performed the surgery for fistula should administer the follow-up care, seeing the patient at weekly intervals. Regardless of the extent of the surgery, it is seldom necessary to see a patient in the office more than two or three times.

REFERENCES

Goodsall, D. H., and Miles, W. E., Diseases of the Anus and Rectum. Part 1. Longman's, London, 1900.

Hanley, P. H., Anorectal abscess fistula. Surg. Clin. North Am., 58:495, 1978.

Parks, A. G., Gordon, P. H., and Hardcastle, J. D., A classification of fistula-in-ano. Br. J. Surg., 63:1–12, 1976.

CHAPTER 7

ANAL FISSURE

INTRODUCTION

Anal fissures are linear ulcers in the anal canal that usually occur in the midline posteriorly. They may, however, occur in the midline anteriorly, chiefly in women. They are seldom found laterally. The typical fissure is an ellipitically shaped ulcer with a "punched-out" appearance. It is generally pink, but the base frequently penetrates to the level of the pale, circular fibers of the internal sphincter muscle. Fissures are among the most painful lesions occurring in the anal canal. They are slightly more common in men and are seldom multiple.

PATHOLOGY

A fissure is not identical to an abrasion. Abrasions may occur anywhere along the circumference of the anal verge and usually result from the passage of large, dry stool. They are common in individuals who do not maintain an adequate diet, good bowel habits, and proper anal hygiene. Fissures are apt to occur in the tense or "ulcer-type" individual. This type of person is likely to have anal spasm, irregular bowel habits, and an improper diet.

Fissures may begin as a painful abrasion, which in turn causes anal spasm, especially in the tense individual. Repeated irritation and constant spasm prevent drainage and healing of the abrasions, resulting in an ulcer. This ulcer is actually an acute fissure and is easily curable at this stage.

The next stage in the development of a fissure is characterized by deeper penetration of the skin and inflammation caused by poor drainage of the anal crypts. There is slight edema of the skin distal to the ulcer and swelling of the adjacent papillae. The ulcer can now be classified as a subacute fissure but is still potentially curable without surgery.

If neglected, the chronic ulcer will penetrate the full thickness of skin lining the anal canal, exposing the fibers of the internal sphincter muscle. There is an associated skin tag of variable size and an enlarged papilla, and other papillae may be prominent. It is thought that direct involvement of the internal sphincter muscle by the ulcer causes pain, which produces prolonged spasm and its associated side effects. The prolonged spasm of the sphincter muscle often prompts the patient to use stool softeners to keep the bowel movements soft or liquid. Soft stools severely limit the amount of exercise the sphincter muscle receives, and when deprived of this exercise for a period of months the normal muscle of the lower border of the internal sphincter is replaced by fibrous tissue and anal stenosis of a variable degree is inevitable. It is not entirely understood why the contraction process affects the lower border of the internal sphincter or why the entire circumference is involved.

Chronic fissures can also cause subcutaneous abscesses because the infection may not remain localized in the anal crypts and in the ulcer itself. Attempts to expell a firm stool through a contracted anal canal can cause abrasions, which then foster the spread of infection.

DIAGNOSIS

In 95 per cent of patients, chronic fissure may be correctly diagnosed by the history alone. There is pain during bowel movements and it may last for varying periods of time, depending on the severity of the fissure. A trace of blood is noted on the toilet tissue, and frequently the patient has been taking laxatives or mineral oil to keep the stools soft in an effort to avoid pain. The history of discomfort covers a period from months to years. The patient is generally young and in good health.

By spreading the skin of both buttocks carefully with the patient in the knee-chest position, the punched-out, small pink or reddish ulcer is seen in the anal canal, along with the characteristic skin tag. Because of anal spasm and pain, it is seldom possible for the patient to relax sufficiently for the examiner to see the entire fissure or the enlarged papilla at the dentate line.

Fissures are extremely painful, and in some patients the discomfort may last an entire day after a bowel movement. Therefore, it is necessary in some cases to rule out the presence of an abscess. In the female patient, if the small finger cannot be introduced into the anal canal because of pain or contraction, the index finger can be introduced into the vagina and the anal canal can be properly examined. The thumb of the same hand or the fingers of the other hand are used for counterpressure to evaluate the intervening structures. In the male patient, if there is significant doubt as to the presence of an abscess, it may be necessary to inject the base of the ulcer with a local anesthetic before attempting to insert the examining finger. Fortunately, this is seldom necessary.

In dealing with fissures of this severity, I usually use the small-caliber pediatric sigmoidoscope to confirm the diagnosis. If this is not possible, I explain the situation to the patient and urge that further examination and treatment be performed utilizing complete local anesthesia. In such patients a stricturotomy must be performed, and, after gradually working the scope into the anal canal, an internal sphincterotomy is often necessary before a large enough anoscope can be introduced for proper examination.

Differential Diagnosis

A chronic anal fissure can rarely be mistaken for anything else. The triad of skin tag, ulcer, and enlarged papilla is inevitably present. The most characteristic features are the severe pain and the normal appearance of skin immediately surrounding the fissure. There is no thickening, infiltration, or undermining, and the skin is not moth-eaten in appearance. Thickening of the surrounding skin occurs only in the presence of abscess formation. This is rarely seen in fissures and when present is easily recognized for what it is—a subcutaneous abscess. If in doubt about the diagnosis, do not hesitate to repeat the history and examination.

Tumors, especially the more rare types, may sometimes pose a diagnostic problem. A patient 62 years of age presented with pain and slight bleeding at bowel movements, and a small protrusion at the anal verge. Examination revealed a superficial fissure and a firm skin tag at the anal verge in the midline posteriorly. This had the appearance of a chronic fissure with skin tag. However, the skin tag was firm and not soft, as seen in fissures. It was not an external thrombotic hemorrhoid or abscess. The only firm benign lesion protruding from the anus would be a prolapsing enlarged papilla, and this would be recognized by its attachment at the dentate line. Although I did not suspect malignancy, I suspected the presence of something in addition to fissure. A wide excision of the fissure and tag was performed. The laboratory report indicated a very low-grade adenocarcinoma arising in the anal ducts. Since all the disease appeared to be well below the dentate line, it was decided to wait one or two months before advising radical surgery. However, the tumor recurred within two months and a Miles abdominoperineal resection was performed.

An ulcerating adenocarcinoma of the lower portion of the rectum may involve the anal canal and can indeed protrude from the anus. By the same token, a squamous-cell tumor of the anal canal or perianal region may extend upward and involve the dentate line and lower rectum. Both of these tumors may be present as an ulceration and could conceivably be mistaken for fissure. The infiltration and elevated borders of these tumors, in contradistinction to the clear, punched-out appearance of a fissure, should prompt the examiner to perform a biopsy with local anesthesia.

Troublesome bleeding in performing a biopsy can be avoided if a small wedge of tissue from the elevated border of the lesion is obtained. Trauma to normal tissue should be avoided, and hemostasis can easily be obtained by coagulating the raw area with the Hyfrecator and needle-point electrode. A tissue specimen approximately 2 to 4 mm in diameter is sufficient for examination. Since the biopsy specimen constitutes only a portion of the tumor's volume, digital examination is necessary to demonstrate its actual size and involvement.

Anorectal fissures associated with *Crohn's disease* may complicate the diagnosis, since this disease may be limited to the anorectal area for periods up to 10 years before other portions of the bowel have demonstrable lesions. However, the ulcers are larger than the usual fissure, may show undermining of the skin, tend to be multiple, and have no predilection for the midline posteriorly. The skin around the ulcers tends to be thickened, and there is a tendency to abscess formation. The mucosa of the rectum is usually normal, which may confuse the examiner, who expects proctitis or colitis in association with Crohn's disease. Biopsy of the edge of one of the ulcers may show granulomas, but just as often it does not; therefore Crohn's disease remains a clinical diagnosis.

Ulcerative colitis may mimic fissure in the anorectal area, tempting the physician to perform fissurectomy. This is generally the wrong thing to do, since the wounds may never heal and continence, already compromised by the colitis, may be lost. Conservative management is always indicated in these cases. Diagnosis is easy because of the history of ulcerative colitis.

Proctoscopic examination, barium enema and/or colonoscopy with stool examinations, and mucosal biopsy will verify the diagnosis of ulcerative colitis, while ruling out disorders such as amebic dysentery.

Idiopathic pruritis ani may present abrasions, superficial fissures, and occasional subcutaneous abscesses because of infection initiated by the trauma of scratching. The characteristic thickened, lichenified skin and a history of severe itching that is worse at night are diagnostic. Pruritis ani usually occurs in the tense individual and is very common. I refer to it as a "space-age" disease, although it is more of a nuisance than a disease. It is primarily a medical condition, and surgical procedures only add to the suffering by causing scars, contraction, and occasional leakage of stool. I see 10 to 15 such patients each day.

Blood disorders may cause atypical deep indolent ulcerations at the anal area. Leukemia is one of the most common offenders. This is relatively rare and can be diagnosed by general physical examination, blood counts, bone marrow examinations, and similar investigations.

Tuberculosis of the anal area is seldom seen today. I have not seen this disease in the past 20 years and have never seen a primary tuberculous ulcer of the anorectal area. It is always secondary to pulmonary tuberculosis or to tubercular disease higher in the intestinal tract. Tuberculous ulcers are large and nonpainful, with undermining of the skin edges. The ulcers are characteristic in that they are shallow and nodular at the base. These signs, in addition to the absence of fistulas, serve to differentiate tuberculous ulcers from Crohn's disease.

A clinical diagnosis is easily made in the presence of proven pulmonary tuberculosis. Bacteriologic and histologic diagnoses are more difficult. Scrapings of the ulcers for smear and culture with guinea pig inoculation will confirm the diagnosis. Biopsy for histologic examination, however, may or may not show the typical appearance of tuberculosis.

It is doubtful that *syphilis* of the anus could be confused with fissure, even though the chancre that is the primary stage of syphilis resembles a fissure during the very early stage of development. History and bacteriologic studies should suffice to confirm the diagnosis.

TREATMENT

Chronic fissures require surgery that often involves cutting various portions of the internal sphincter muscle. There is no satisfactory nonsurgical treatment for this condition. While surgery is mandatory, some patients suffer from various degrees of anal incontinence following even the most skillfully performed operation. Thus a conservative approach to management seems justified.

Treatment of fissure is relatively simple if a correct diagnosis is made. Furthermore, many afflictions involving the anal canal are self-limited. This is not always true with fissures, since many acute fissures may become chronic if not properly managed. Anal abrasions may heal spontaneously, although it is better to initiate a course of treatment if the patient seeks advice.

The treatments for anal abrasions and acute and subacute fissures are identical. This requires a general approach. Obesity, poor dietary or bowel habits, inadequate anal hygiene, any organic or functional disease, must be corrected. A high-residue and high-vitamin diet is usually indicated. Daily sources of vitamin C and whole-grain breads and cereals are especially important. Slender patients with diarrhea do better on concentrated foods such as bananas, potatoes, rice, eggs, and meat. Psyllium hydrophilic mucilloid preparations (Metamucil) may help thicken the stool. Development of a regular bowel habit—usually one stool after breakfast each morning—is encouraged. The anal area must be cleansed thoroughly after each bowel movement with cotton soaked in witch hazel. I have seen many patients do well on this regime alone. Obese patients may need additional bulk, such as Metamucil, for constipation or diarrhea and to help decrease their appetite, which will help them lose weight.

The local treatment is quite simple. Patients are instructed to apply an ointment containing 5 per cent sulfathiazole and 1 per cent benzocaine to the anal canal several times a day using the index finger covered by a finger cot. This provides a soothing effect, and promotes healing and gentle dilatation of the sphincter muscles. Analgesics can be administered if necessary.

Most abrasions and acute fissures heal in a few weeks. The subacute fissure may require several months; in fact, not all subacute fissures will heal. Some will progress to the chronic stage and require surgery. Some fissures heal temporarily only to recur in a few months to a year. Unless the fissure becomes chronic, conservative treatment is indicated. The physician must keep the patient informed as to the appearance of the fissure. Conversely, the patient must keep the physician apprised of his condition, since the question of how long to continue conservative treatment depends on the amount of discomfort experienced.

Surgery is the only cure for a chronic fissure. While the surgical principles have remained the same, the methods have changed. The traditional method of operation for fissure, the posterior sphincterotomy, was improved by Eisenhammer, who advised a lateral sphincterotomy incision with excision of the fissure itself posteriorly. In this way the anal crypts were not excised. Many surgeons now view lateral sphincterotomy as the only treatment for anal fissure, except in the presence of a large, troublesome skin tag or an enlarged papilla, in which case these are excised.

The great majority of patients who need surgery for fissure will have additional problems such as hemorrhoids. It is thus logical and desirable to combine a sphincterotomy with hemorrhoidectomy (Fig. 7–1 and 7–2). In fact, a sphincterotomy alone in a patient with medium to large hemorrhoids will

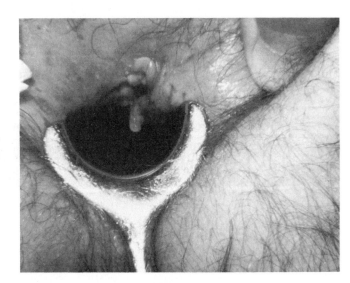

Figure 7–1. Depicts chronic fissure that is treated by lateral sphincterotomy and excision of crypts, hemorrhoids and fissure.

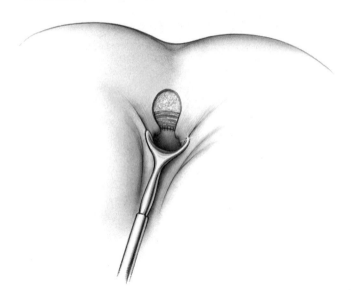

Figure 7–2. Wound remaining after total excision.

predispose to the prolapse of the internal hemorrhoids due to postsurgical relaxation of the anal canal.

My preference when dealing with chronic anal fissure is to perform a partial internal sphincterotomy laterally. A radial incision is made just distal to the dentate line and extending just beyond the anal verge. The wound is separated with a small hemostat, and the white fibers of the internal sphincter muscle are identified. The intersphincteric groove is seen and palpated. Just distal to the groove are the pink to reddish fleshy fibers of the external sphincter. It is easy to identify the constrictive band causing the anal contraction. Only enough of the lower border of the internal sphincter is cut to allow insertion of a large Hill-Ferguson retractor. *Under no circumstances should the muscle be cut higher than the dentate line.* The skin incision is closed with interrupted catgut sutures, and the operation is completed by excising the skin tag and fissure as well as the enlarged papilla (Fig. 7–3).

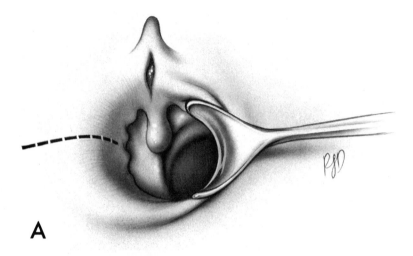

A

Figure 7–3. A, Type of fissure treated by limited excision.

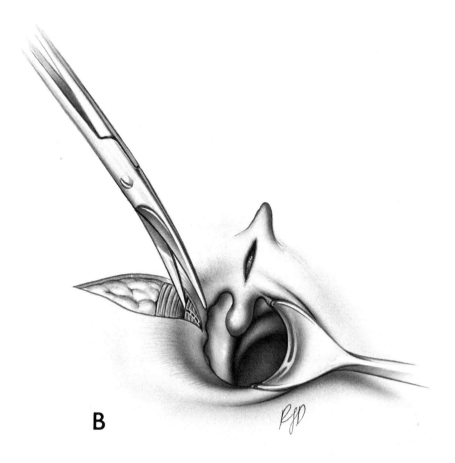

B

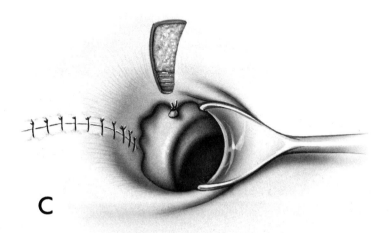

C

Figure 7–3. *Continued. B*, Partial internal sphincterotomy. *C,* Appearance of remaining wounds.

POSTOPERATIVE CARE

It is generally advisable to make postoperative care as simple as possible. When this principle is followed, patients are more apt to comply with instructions. However, the amount of care needed is directly proportional to the extent of the surgery and may vary from no special care or disability to 12 days of rest with special precautions relative to bowel movements.

When partial internal sphincterotomy alone is performed, the patient leaves the office and may return to work immediately, although usually the operative day is lost from work. The patient is given an analgesic, stops taking laxatives or stool softeners, and should resume forming normal stools immediately. The patient returns to the office within seven days for a routine examination. It is rare, but these wounds can become infected, and for that reason careful follow-up is necessary.

REFERENCES

Eisenhammer, S., The evaluation of internal sphincterotomy operation with special reference to anal fissure. Surg. Gynecol Obstet., 109:583, 1959.

Gathright, J. B., Personal communication, 1982.

Goldberg, S. M., Gordon, P. H., and Nivatvongs, S., Essentials of Anorectal Surgery. Philadelphia, J. B. Lippincott, 1980, p. 98.

Goligher, J. C., Surgery of the Anus, Rectum and Colon, 4th ed. Baillière Tindall, London, 1980.

CHAPTER 8

HEMORRHOIDS

INTRODUCTION

Hemorrhoids, or piles, are enlarged or varicose veins at the rectal outlet. Many children and most adults have them. They are the most frequent cause of rectal bleeding. Although one of the most common anorectal diseases, hemorrhoidal disease is frequently overtreated, both medically and surgically. While I do not know of a single patient who has died of hemorrhoids, I do know of some who have died as a result of improper treatment.

Patients with hemorrhoidal disease can be divided into two groups. The asymptomatic group, which represents the vast majority of patients, requires no treatment. The symptomatic group of patients present with bleeding, prolapse, external clots, or generalized acute hemorrhoidal disease characterized by swelling of variable degree of all or a part of the hemorrhoidal plexus.

CLASSIFICATION

Anatomy is important in understanding the nature, symptoms, and treatment of hemorrhoids.

Internal hemorrhoids occur above the anorectal line and are covered by mucosa. They are supplied by nerves of the autonomic nervous system and are therefore insensitive to painful stimuli. Thus internal hemorrhoids may be present without warning symptoms of pain. *External hemorrhoids* are situated below the anorectal line and are covered by skin. They are innervated by the inferior hemorrhoidal nerve, which makes them exceedingly sensitive to pain. Although the two types can be recognized easily, they are in close proximity, which often makes separate treatment of each type difficult. *Mixed hemorrhoids,* or combined internal and external hemorrhoids, are seen frequently. In symptomatic cases mixed hemorrhoids are associated with various degrees of prolapse of the anal canal. They require surgery if they are to be eradicated completely.

Like many other clinical entities, hemorrhoids can be graded on the basis of their severity (Fig. 8–1). The grading of hemorrhoids has significance in guiding treatment (see p. 96). Internal and external hemorrhoids should be graded separately and treated accordingly. For example, a patient may have

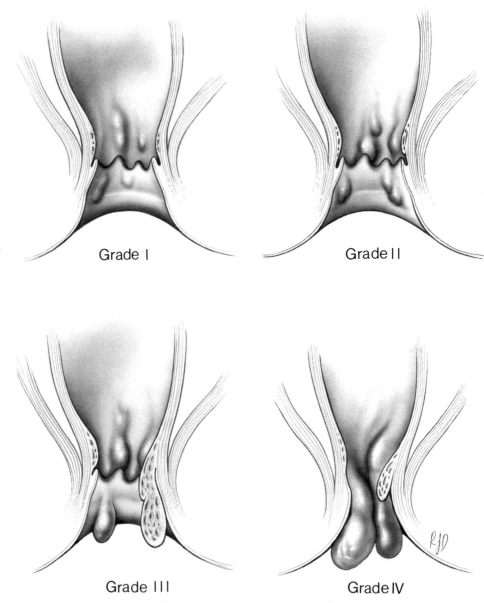

Figure 8–1. Grades of hemorrhoids.

very small (grade I) internal and larger (grade II to IV) external hemorrhoids or vice versa. Small grade I internal and external hemorrhoids are usually asymptomatic and should require no specific treatment. Unfortunately, some patients with grade I hemorrhoids have unusually thin skin and will have some bleeding and irritation at times due to abrasions. Some of these patients will not or cannot comprehend the importance of a holistic approach to medicine in which improvement of general health by weight control, proper diet, and anal hygiene will correct the problem. In such cases, even surgery will be followed by poor healing. Such patients will continue to challenge every method of management.

Grade II internal and external hemorrhoids may have slight bleeding, although they do not prolapse. These may be occasional small, thrombotic external hemorrhoids. Injection or rubber band treatment of internal hemorrhoids and excision of thrombotic external hemorrhoids should suffice.

Grade III internal hemorrhoids may bleed and protrude at bowel movement but can easily be replaced, whereas grade IV internal hemorrhoids bleed at bowel movement and show constant protrusion that cannot be replaced. Grades III and IV external hemorrhoids require surgery for cure.

DIAGNOSIS

Many patients experience large external hemorrhoids and even mild to moderate prolapse of internal hemorrhoids without complaint. As stated previously, asymptomatic hemorrhoids do not require treatment.

Thrombosis of external hemorrhoids is characterized by a sudden lump at the anal verge or in the immediate perianal area. Such lumps may vary in size from a few millimeters to several inches in diameter. These lumps are due to the rupture of one or more subcutaneous veins, allowing blood to escape into the subcutaneous tissue and causing much pain. They eventually become clots and are either absorbed gradually or break through the overlying skin, thereby allowing the old blood to escape and the swelling to recede gradually. The blood clots can be recognized by their sharp delineation from the surrounding tissues and bluish color, which may be seen through the overlying skin. There may be several or many clots with associated swelling and edema. The patient may attempt to push these lumps back into the rectum, but this is impossible because they are merely swollen structures that normally belong on the outside.

Internal hemorrhoids, covered by delicate mucosa, frequently bleed and protrude. Initially the hemorrhoids may protrude only at bowel movement and recede spontaneously or can easily be pushed back into the rectum. However, in time they protrude permanently, and the overlying mucosa creates a "wet anus." Occasionally, prolapsing internal hemorrhoids become gangrenous because of a contracted anal sphincter, or they may be associated with a generalized swelling of the external hemorrhoids causing acute hemorrhoidal disease. The appearance of acute hemorrhoidal disease is startling, but inspection and digital examination help to differentiate the condition from abscess, perianal cellulitis, or other infections.

Acute hemorrhoidal disease requires conservative treatment, even in the presence of gangrene of some or most of the internal hemorrhoids. In fact, the worse the appearance at this stage, the more important it is to treat the condition conservatively to avoid postoperative bleeding (see p. 101).

TREATMENT

Acute attacks of hemorrhoids are frequently triggered by straining at stool or trauma during childbirth. What is not generally known is that with the exception of chronic or constantly prolapsed internal hemorrhoids and the very rare "arterial" hemorrhoids, both of which require definitive treatment, hemorrhoidal disease is self-limited.

With few exceptions, complications will not occur if the formation of dry, firm stools is prevented. The diet should therefore include bulk. The anus should be cleaned thoroughly after each bowel movement with tissue followed by cotton soaked in witch hazel. Soothing ointments or lotions such as hydrocortisone acetate and pramoxine hydrochloride (Proctofoam-HC) are sometimes indicated. In other words, skillful neglect with symptomatic treatment will, in the vast majority of instances, allow the patient to recover from the acute attack. However, one must be practical and diplomatic. The patient who experiences repeated attacks of hemorrhoidal disease will demand a definitive method of treatment.

Modern local anesthesia has made it possible to avoid hospitalization in the treatment of most anorectal diseases; however, in practice more and more complete hemorrhoidectomies are being performed in the hospital to minimize nervous tension on the part of the patient and to avoid potential medicolegal problems. Fortunately, the vast majority of patients suffering from hemorrhoids may be treated by simple and safe alternative therapies that can be performed on an outpatient basis.

INJECTION THERAPY

Hemorrhoids are treated only when they are symptomatic. If they are small, do not protrude, and exhibit bleeding (grade II), sclerosing therapy with 5 per cent phenol in almond oil may suffice (Fig. 8–2). The purpose is not to inject the solution into the veins but to inject it submucosally, with the expectation that the resulting inflammatory reaction will create fibrosis of the tissue and "shrink" the hemorrhoid. Sclerotherapy requires neither anesthesia nor hospitalization.

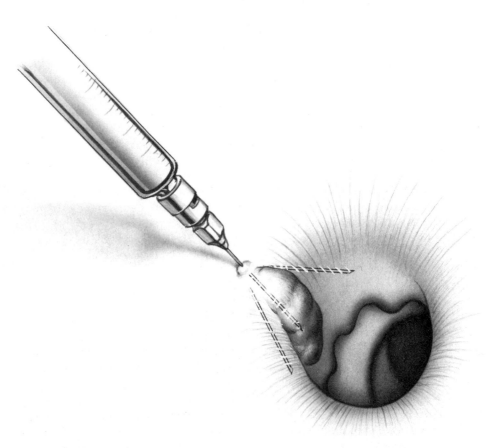

Figure 8–2. Injecting local anesthetic agent prior to excision of external thrombotic hemorrhoid.

RUBBER BAND LIGATION

Larger protruding internal hemorrhoids (grades III and IV) are treated by the rubber band ligation method, except in obese women with short anal canals. In such patients, it is difficult to maintain reduction. Figure 8–3 shows the rubber band placed externally merely to demonstrate the method.

A rubber band is placed around the hemorrhoid with the aid of an ingenious instrument invented by Barron. Anesthesia is not necessary. The internal hemorrhoid is choked off and sloughs away with the rubber band in a few days (Fig. 8–4). Because major hemorrhage from slough is a possibility requiring electrocautery as an emergency procedure, larger hemorrhoids are treated two or more times rather than choking off too much tissue at once. One hemorrhoid is ligated at a time, with the procedure repeated at 3-week intervals until all of them have been removed. Usually there are three internal hemorrhoids to be treated. Often after such treatment, any external hemorrhoids resolve spontaneously. If not, they can be treated by simple excision in the office under local anesthesia.

Rubber band ligation of hemorrhoids may cause complications. The rubber band must not be placed near or below the sensitive anorectal line because of the possibility of causing severe pain. If there is any pain after placing the band, I immediately move the band so that it does not encroach on the anorectal line or produce tension on the tissues.

Sometimes in moving or removing the rubber bands the mucosa is torn and bleeds. In such cases, if feasible, I immediately place another band so as to incorporate the bleeding portion of the hemorrhoid. If this is not possible, I attempt to fulgurate the laceration; and if this does not suffice, I use complete local anesthesia, making it possible to suture the injured tissue.

The rubber band ligation of hemorrhoids will leave a rather large, raw area when the band sloughs off. This raw area tends to persist for up to six weeks after treatment, and therefore the possibility of secondary bleeding persists beyond the usual 8 to 12 days following conventional hemorrhoidectomy. This is probably due to the fact that the raw area or ulcer has no drainage. The patient must be warned against the use of enemas or straining at stool during this six-week period.

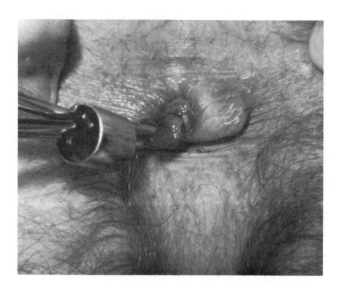

Figure 8–3. Application of the rubber band externally.

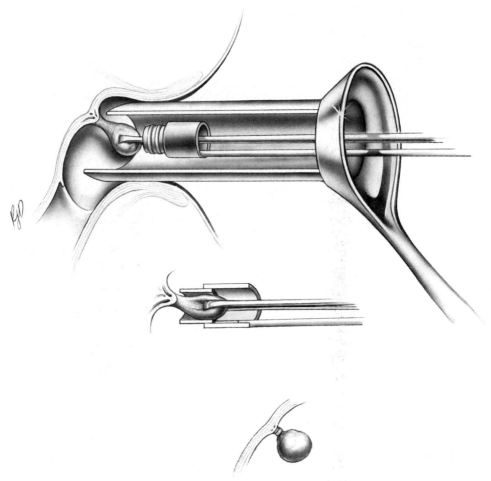

Figure 8–4. Barron or rubber band ligation.

I sometimes fulgurate small bleeding internal hemorrhoids that do not respond to injection therapy and are too small for the effective use of a rubber band. In such cases it is important to avoid fulgurating an area wider than 3 to 4 mm and deeper than the full thickness of mucosa to avoid secondary bleeding.

ACUTE HEMORRHOIDAL DISEASE

Acute hemorrhoidal disease (Fig. 8–5), characterized by acute prolapse of the anal canal with thrombophlebitis of the hemorrhoidal plexus and, occasionally, by necrosis or gangrene (Fig. 8–6), is usually best treated conservatively with hot or cold compresses and administration of mineral oil by mouth to ensure easy bowel movements. The condition will often resolve itself. When seen within the first 24 to 48 hours, injection of a local anesthetic with hyaluronidase (Wydase) will occasionally reduce the swelling completely and make immediate hemorrhoidectomy possible (Fig. 8–7). This is seldom necessary, however, since it is far safer to use conservative measures such as pain-relieving ointment and analgesics until the acute inflammatory process has subsided. By this time, the patient often feels so much better that surgery becomes optional.

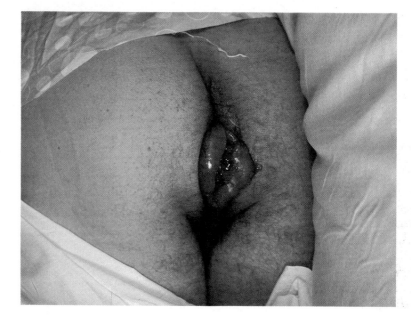

Figure 8–5. Acute hemorrhoidal disease.

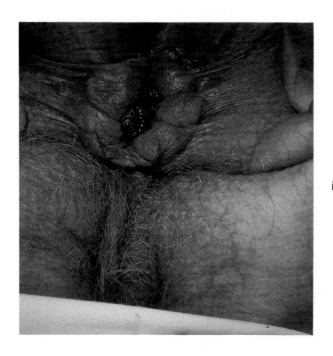

Figure 8–6. Gangrenous internal hemorrhoids.

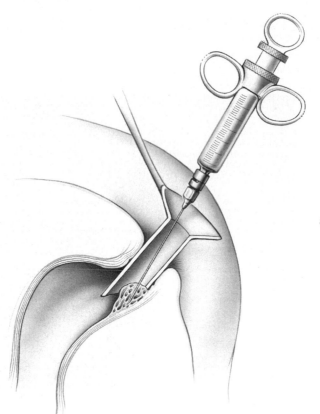

Figure 8–7. Sclerotherapy for internal hemorrhoids.

THROMBOTIC EXTERNAL HEMORRHOID

Perhaps the most frequent anorectal surgical condition encountered in the office is a thrombotic external hemorrhoid. After introducing a small amount of anesthetic solution around and beneath the thrombosis, the clot can be removed with a simple elliptical incision (Figs. 8–8 to 8–10). Often the wound margins fall together after the clot is removed. Usually nothing is needed to control bleeding, and primary union follows. If bleeding occurs, it can be controlled by fulguration, or the vessel—usually a small vein—can be ligated with triple 0 chromic catgut. A small pressure dressing can be used to prevent development of another thrombus. If in doubt, the skin wounds may be easily closed with triple 0 chromic catgut (Figs. 8–11 to 8–13).

In excision of a thrombotic external hemorrhoid, be certain of your diagnosis and remove only the thrombus with an elliptical, relatively narrow segment of overlying skin so that when the operation is completed, the skin margins fall together and a pressure dressing will permit primary healing. The result should appear as a simple linear incision, and the surrounding tissue should be flat and free of edema. If edema and generalized swelling are present, chances are that the condition is thrombophlebitis or acute hemorrhoidal disease and not a simple thrombus. Cutting into edematous tissue in such instances will not relieve the pain and frequently will compound the problem. If in doubt, use conservative measures. I will occasionally remove more than one thrombus or even a cluster of thrombi at one time, but I try to make sure of the diagnosis before proceeding with treatment. Hemostasis must be complete before the patient leaves the office.

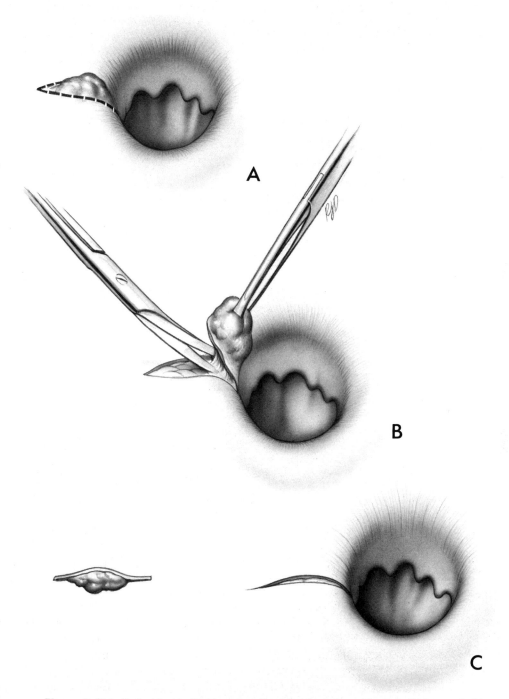

Figure 8–8. *A,* Dotted line indicates area of incision for external thrombotic hemorrhoid. *B,* Excision is begun. *C,* Excision is completed.

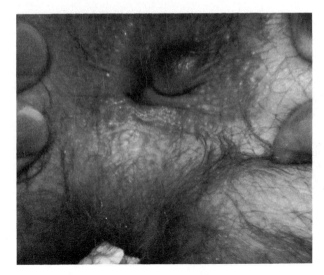

Figure 8–9. Thrombotic external hemorrhoid.

Figure 8–10. Specimen after excision.

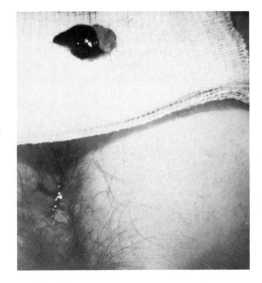

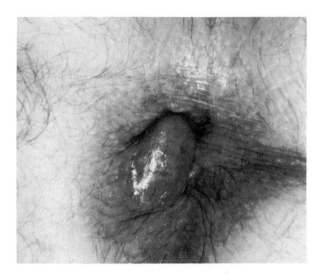

Figure 8–11. Large thrombotic external hemorrhoid.

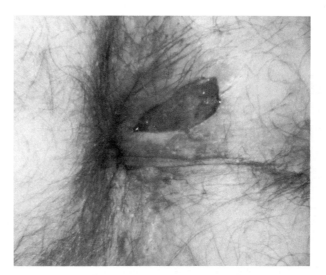

Figure 8–12. Wound after excision.

HYPERTROPHIED PAPILLAE

An occasional patient will have only an enlarged papilla that may even protrude from the anal canal (Figs. 8–14 and 8–15). Excision of the papilla will relieve the patient's symptoms.

HEMORRHOIDECTOMY

Selection of Patients. The technic of complete hemorrhoidectomy in the office is easy, but the selection of patients is important. There are certain patients who will not or cannot cope with postoperative discomfort at home. Others will develop urinary retention. Performing extensive office procedures on neurotic, highly emotional or elderly patients should be avoided.

Some surgeons place great emphasis on age in selecting patients for hemorrhoidectomy, believing that individuals 60 years of age or older are apt to heal poorly and will not be properly relieved of their symptoms. However, with the use of local anesthesia, I have found that when the true indications for surgery are present, age alone is not a contraindication. I have operated

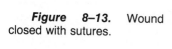

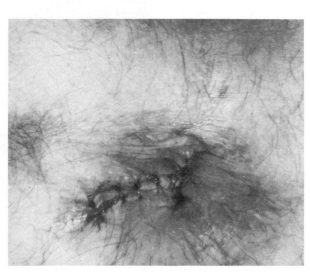

Figure 8–13. Wound closed with sutures.

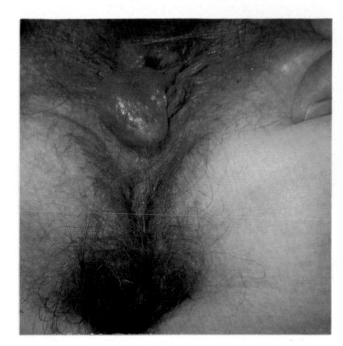

Figure 8–14. Papilla.

Figure 8–15. Papilla.

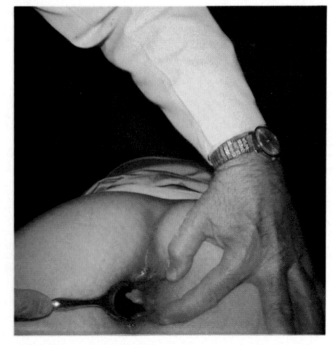

on patients of all age groups and shall continue to do so. In fact, many older patients are less apprehensive and tolerate the surgery better than younger patients.

The patients I am concerned about, regardless of age, are those with a generally poor health profile. They are usually obese, suffering from cardiovascular and/or metabolic problems, and taking several medications, including insulin, aspirin, and anticoagulants. Caution and conservatism are essential in the effective treatment of hemorrhoids in these patients. However, there are exceptions to every rule, and the usual treatment may be administered if indicated and if it is feasible to interrupt the existing therapy such as anticoagulant therapy. It should be emphasized, however, that the vast majority of these medically compromised patients require general medical care more urgently than they need proctologic treatment.

Once in several hundred cases, a patient with normal hematologic studies (including coagulation profile) will bleed profusely from hemorrhoids. Sometimes transfusions are required. Usually such hemorrhoids are of the spongy or "arterial" type, as identified by Buie. Hospitalization is required in such cases.

Other indications for hospital surgery include huge hemorrhoids associated with severe protrusion in which the lowermost portion of the rectal lining is "turned inside out," and the coexistence of hemorrhoids with other extensive rectal problems such as deep fistulas.

Technic. Hemorrhoids swell slightly, especially when a person is standing, coughing, or straining, and in this manner supplement the function of the anal sphincter in prohibiting the involuntary escape of flatus or stool. It is for this reason that if continence is to be preserved, a modern hemorrhoidectomy does not involve removal of all hemorrhoids of the anorectal line.

Many patients present with a scarred, contracted, almost useless anal canal that is the result of radical hemorrhoidectomy. These patients complain of diarrhea and attribute the problem to a spastic colon. They frequently state that they have "colitis," and it is only through careful questioning that they will admit their inability to control flatus or stool. These unfortunate patients had their operations many years ago, have suffered much psychic trauma, and have good reason for their spastic or nervous colons.

Usually there are three and sometimes more groups of hemorrhoids, and radial incisions are required to remove them (Fig. 8–16A). The surgeon should attempt to save as much normal tissue between the groups as possible.

At the beginning of the operation it is important to start the dissection 1 or 1½ inches distal to the anal verge to prevent skin tags and unhealed granulating areas. By careful dissection the varicosities can be removed down to the muscle. If longitudinal muscle is present, and this is usually a continuation of the internal circular muscle of the bowel, it is left alone. However, in the majority of cases longitudinal muscle is not present or cannot be demonstrated and dissection is carried down to the circular external sphincter muscles. Primary closure with interrupted or running triple 0 chromic catgut is preferred when this can be done without tension (Fig. 8–16B). Sometimes it is necessary to remove the subcutaneous plexus of veins from underneath the preserved anoderm before proceeding with the primary closure; however, one must treat each case individually.

Partial lateral internal sphincterotomy, when performed in patients with a coexisting chronic anal contraction or fissure, is another way to relieve the patient's symptoms and encourage primary healing (see p. 93). This should not be used in very elderly patients or in those suffering from diarrhea.

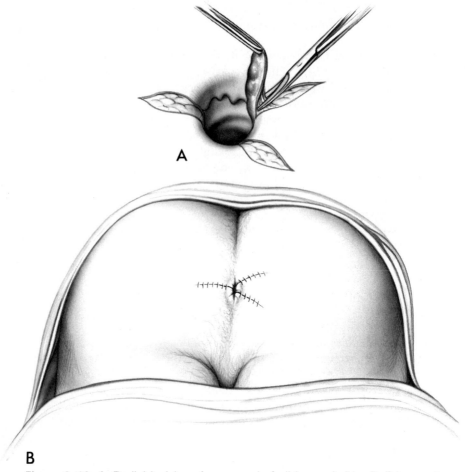

Figure 8–16. *A*, Radial incisions for removal of all hemorrhoids. *B*, Primary closure of wounds.

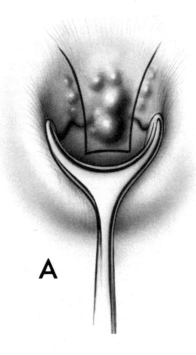

Figure 8–17. *A*, Incision for creating a posterior skin flap.

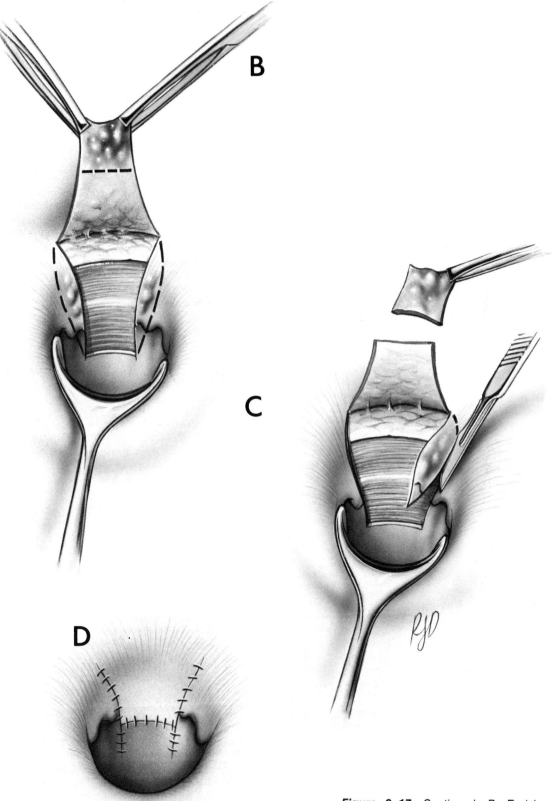

Figure 8–17. *Continued. B,* Excising hemorrhoids from skin flap. *C,* Excising hemorrhoids from either side of skin flap. *D,* Completed skin flap.

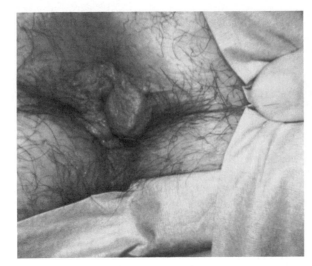

Figure 8–18. Before creating skin flap.

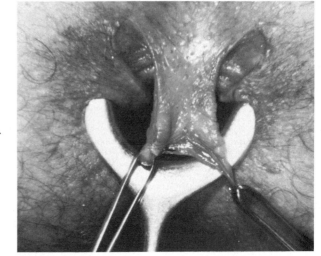

Figure 8–19. The flap.

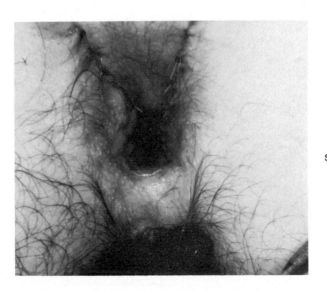

Figure 8–20. Completed skin flap.

Closure. In my opinion, the perfect hemorrhoidectomy has not been devised for all patients. The "closed" method, in which both internal and external components of the hemorrhoidectomy are closed, is attractive and works well in many patients. In my experience, the closed method, unless accompanied with sphincterotomy to avoid sphincter spasm, is associated with a high rate of skin tags and sometimes with fissurelike unhealed areas. The "open" method, in which the external wound is left open, is a safe, effective approach that has stood the test of time. The patients may leave the hospital and resume activities just as quickly as those having the "closed" technic. Since sphincterotomy is performed less frequently, there is less chance of seepage from sphincter impairment. However, patients are also subject to skin tags and poor healing. Enough skin must be excised, as shown in Figure 8–16A, to allow for adequate drainage and to prevent formation of skin tags.

For some unexplainable reason, a wound in the midline posteriorly will heal slowly, but wounds placed close to the midline laterally, such as at the left posterior (11 o'clock) or right posterior (1 o'clock), may not heal at all without further surgery. For this reason I use a posterior sliding skin flap in patients with hemorrhoids involving the entire posterior third of the anorectal area.

Posterior Skin Flap. Two short incisions are made in the skin beginning just beyond the external hemorrhoid on either side of the midline and extending above the dentate line to just above the internal hemorrhoidal area. The incisions should be slanted slightly toward the midline so that the external width is 1½ inches and the inner portion is 1 inch. The intervening hemorrhoids are removed so that normal skin and normal mucosa can be approximated at the dentate line to form a new line at its normal position. Sutures through the mucosa are also anchored to a small bit of the internal sphincter muscle.

After the posterior sliding skin graft is created and before suturing is begun, the internal and external hemorrhoidal tissue lateral to each incision is trimmed away. The skin flap is then approximated to the cut edge of mucosa at the dentate line. This usually requires five or six sutures applied transversely. The mucosa is closed by interrupted or continuous suture, and when the level of the dentate line is reached, the cut edge of skin is united with the lateral edge of the skin flap until the wound is completely closed. A similar closure is accomplished on the opposite side (Figs. 8–17 to 8–20).

The operation is completed by removing hemorrhoids or other disease and tissue that remain laterally or anteriorly.

REFERENCES

Barron, J., Office ligation treatment of hemorrhoids. Dis. Colon Rectum, 6:109, 1963.

Buie, L. A., Practical Proctology. W. B. Saunders Company, Philadelphia, 1938, p. 172.

Ferguson, J. A., Mazier, W. R., Ganchrow, M. I. and Friend, W. G., The closed technique of hemorrhoidectomy. Surgery, 70:480, 1971.

Lord, P. H., Conservative management of hemorrhoids. Part II. Dilatation treatment. Clin. Gastroenterol., 4:601, 1975.

5. Parks, A. G., Hemorrhoidectomy. Surg. Clin. North Am., 45:1305, 1965.

MISCELLANEOUS ANORECTAL DISEASES

IDIOPATHIC PRURITUS ANI

INTRODUCTION

Idiopathic pruritus ani is itching of the skin of the anal canal, perianal, perineal, vulvar, scrotal, and buttocks areas.

Over 50 per cent of pruritus ani at the anal area is categorized as idiopathic because its cause is unknown, although nervous tension may be contributory. Patients almost invariably associate the itching with hemorrhoids. While there may be a short period of relatively mild itching associated with acute hemorrhoidal disease, patients with idiopathic pruritus ani actually have few or no hemorrhoids. Idiopathic pruritus ani is primarily a medical condition, and meddlesome surgery such as removal of crypts and small hemorrhoids adds to the suffering of these patients by producing side effects such as seepage. I have seen patients with mucosal prolapse and even procidentia that occurred as a direct result of surgical attempts to remove all or most of the itching skin. Radical surgery practically always removes the normal supports of the rectum at the anorectal line.

PATHOLOGY

There are two types of idiopathic pruritus ani: dry and moist (Figs. 9–1 and 9–2). The skin may be hyperemic, thickened, and lichenified. Scratching may produce abrasions, excoriations, and secondary infections such as pustules or abscesses. Thickening of the dermal layer of the skin (acanthosis) and lymphocytic infiltration of the perivascular tissues resembling neurodermatitis have been shown to characterize the condition.

DIAGNOSIS

The physician's primary responsibility in the diagnosis is to rule out serious disease or other conditions requiring specific treatment. Systemic and local disease must be excluded. Neoplasms are discussed elsewhere (Chap. 15). Diabetes and renal disease occasionally cause itching and thickening of

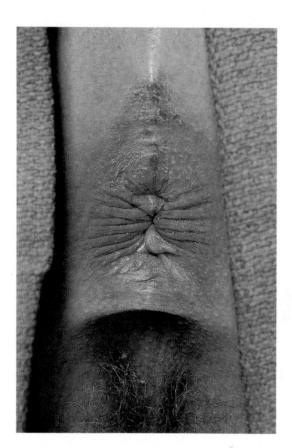

Figure 9–1. Idiopathic pruritus ani (dry).

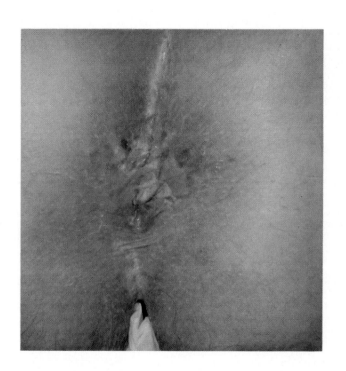

Figure 9–2. Idiopathic pruritus ani (moist).

the skin, but lichenification with variable thickening of the skin is practically pathognomonic of idiopathic pruritus ani. In early cases the skin is a greyish-white color and the thickening may not be grossly evident. However, as the condition progresses, thickening of the skin becomes more evident while the whitish color is always present.

Dermatologic diseases can occur anywhere in the skin and include psoriasis, lichen planus, contact dermatitis, primary fungal and yeast infections, allergies to food and drugs including antibiotics, and acanthosis nigricans, which Buie has associated with the possibility of cancer higher in the bowel. Their detection may require the aid of a dermatologist. In vitiligo (Fig. 9–3), the loss of pigment results in an almost white color. However, vitiligo cannot be confused with idiopathic pruritus ani because the appearance is distinctive and there is no itching. Kraurosis (Fig. 9–4) of the skin at the anus, which some believe is a premalignant lesion, is also a white color, but it is usually localized to a small area with such striking thickening that it seems to invite excisional biopsy. With experience, the clinician will develop the ability to gauge the degree of disease. There are no two cases exactly similar, yet the dermatologist and proctologist who see these patients each day recognize them in a moment.

For the most part, fungus and yeasts, except for Actinomyces and Monilia *(Candida albicans)*, are secondary invaders. Primary fungal infection due to Epidermophyton appears as raised circular frost-like lesions that resemble ringworm. Actinomycosis is rare and characterized by draining sinuses and deep inflammation. The fungus is easily identified on bacteriologic examination of the discharge. Yeast infection (Fig. 9–5) is usually due to extension from monilial infection in the vagina. The lesion caused by Monilia looks as though a fine, granular, moist pink powder were applied in a thin layer at the anal area. Nothing in its appearance suggests the need for biopsy.

Although biopsy of skin is not often performed to diagnose idiopathic pruritus ani, it is necessary where neoplasm is suspected. If anything unusual is noted, such as a nodule or a localized thickening of skin or subcutaneous

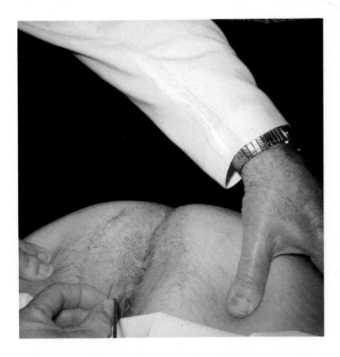

Figure 9–3. Vitiligo.

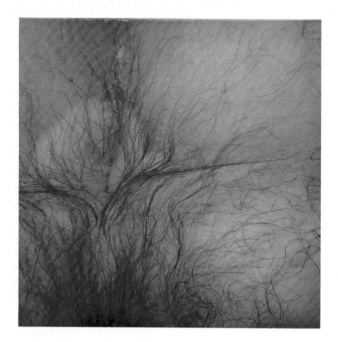

Figure 9–4. Kraurosis.

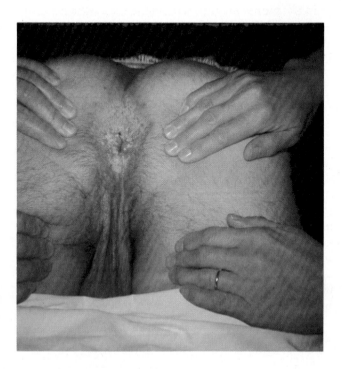

Figure 9–5. Yeast infection.

tissue, an excisional biopsy or a limited incisional biopsy can easily be performed in the office using local anesthesia. The mere presence of idiopathic pruritus ani does not mean that a general investigation need not be conducted. Biopsy, especially if the condition is extensive, can be done at another visit depending on convenience, expediency, and other factors.

TREATMENT

Ice compresses can help stop itching temporarily. Sitz baths and good anal hygiene may be of help in controlling symptoms. Local application of Cortifoam may provide temporary and even permanent relief in some cases of idiopathic pruritus ani, especially the moist type. For the dry type, a nongreasy ointment such as 1 per cent methylprednisone (Medrol) is effective. It is good to vary the type of medication used. Since itching is characteristically worse at night, mild sedation on a temporary basis may help break the cycle of itch, scratch, and itch. Yeasts and fungi are secondary invaders, and general treatment therefore only removes part of the problem. Although dyes are messy, Castellani's paint is effective for the secondary invaders. Mycostatin powder and Whitfield's ointment may also be used for yeasts and fungi.

A totally effective treatment for idiopathic pruritus ani has yet to be found. Here again, the concept of holistic medicine must be applied. Tension and stress will not disappear—it is how we respond to them that is important. Stress can be reduced and general physical and mental health can be improved by maintaining good eating habits and following a balanced program of exercise, weight control, and recreation.

Do not promise a cure but reassure the patient that although the condition is chronic, it is not premalignant. Follow the patient closely to ensure proper management until the patient gains enough confidence to continue the treatment himself. The patient must know and expect the exacerbations that characterize this disease. Many of my patients have learned to live with their disease, and I see them only for their regular yearly examinations.

HIDRADENITIS SUPPURATIVA

INTRODUCTION

Hidradenitis suppurativa is a relatively rare, chronic inflammatory, multicentric disease of the skin that may occur anywhere in the body but it is especially common in the axillae and under the breasts. It is seen equally in men and women, and is due to infection arising in the apocrine sweat glands. Jackman and McQuarrie found that 32 per cent occurred in the perianal area and buttocks.

Extensive disease manifests itself by nodular swellings and sinuses over one or both buttocks, sometimes extending to perineal, scrotal, and pilonidal areas. It looks more formidable than it really is. Some lesions appear as mere superficial nodules, with only occasional sinuses draining pus.

DIAGNOSIS

Careful examination reveals that there is no connection with the anorectal line and its crypts. The process is relatively superficial, being limited to the skin and subcutaneous tissue. There is a peculiar hobnailed sensation on palpation, and some of the nodules connect with adjacent nodules, with induration of the skin tracts running from one nodule to another. It is easy to mistake hidradenitis suppurativa for a complicated fistula or Crohn's disease on hurried examination. However, abscesses and fistulas due to anorectal disease or Crohn's disease are of greater depth, and probing will usually establish this.

One must first think of the possibility of hidradenitis suppurativa and keep in mind its origin in the apocrine sweat glands. Then the indolent nature of this condition will be fully appreciated. It cannot easily be mistaken for multiple pustules, which are thin-walled skin abscesses. Remember that not all the intradermal nodules of hidradenitis suppurativa contain sinuses or pus, nor do all of them communicate with an adjacent nodule or nodules.

TREATMENT

The treatment for hidradenitis suppurativa is surgery. Any other therapy should be considered ineffective. If no more than 4 square centimeters of one buttock is involved, there should be no hesitation in performing surgery under local anesthesia in an outpatient setting. When there is extensive involvement of buttocks and perineum, regional anesthesia in the hospital should be considered.

After preparation of the skin involved, the operation is begun. It is best to start with a sinus that can be probed and lay that particular area open. Usually the probe can follow the sinus tract to an adjacent sinus or nodule and so on until all sinuses are explored and opened. Any nodule that cannot be probed or does not seem to communicate with an adjacent nodule should be excised. It is easier to cut right down on the nodule and then trim the skin edges in such a manner that it is saucerized and will heal from the inside out. At the completion of the operation, all sinuses should have been opened and all nodules removed. Some of these nodules are entirely intradermal, and it is not necessary to cut into the subcutaneous tissue. Bleeding is controlled by lightly fulgurating opened areas of skin or subcutaneous tissue. The time of the operation should be approximately one-half hour.

Figure 9–6 demonstrates the appearance of the wound after operation for

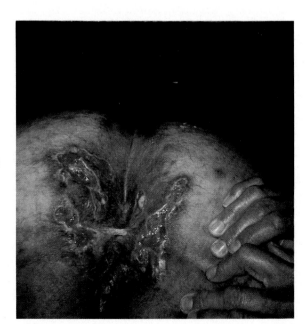

Figure 9–6. Hidradenitis suppurativa after surgery.

a moderately extensive case of hidradenitis suppurativa. The wound will heal nicely with ordinary cleanliness and sitz baths. Diverting colostomy is not necessary, and skin grafts are seldom necessary. Allow several weeks for healing in extensive cases. Any residual or recurrent disease can usually be excised without disability in the office after the original wounds have completely or almost completely healed.

TUBERCULOSIS

INTRODUCTION

Tuberculosis of the anorectal area is a very rare disease. It is still seen in third-world countries, and since it is a possibility that this condition may enter into the differential diagnosis of ulceration at the anorectal area, tuberculosis is included in this discussion.

PATHOLOGY

The bacilli enter the anorectal area through the anal crypts, and for that reason some pathologists think the ulcers at the anorectal area may be multiple. These ulcers tend to join one another to form one large ulcer. Anal tuberculosis will show acanthosis, typical tubercules in the cutis, and epithelioid and giant cells. Caseation necrosis is not seen in the anal area.

DIAGNOSIS

Many years ago, when the disease was more prevalent in the United States, some of the larger clinics found the condition to be more common in the colon than in the anorectal area. In fact, the site most frequently involved was the ileocecal area, and since at that time it was thought that the left colon or the colon distal to the hepatic flexure was seldom involved with tuberculosis, it is possible that many of the patients seen actually had Crohn's disease of the ileocecal area.

Some years ago, when I did see an occasional patient suffering from tuberculosis of the anorectal area, it was of the ulcerative type secondary to pulmonary tuberculosis and involvement of the colon (Fig. 9–7). These ulcers were large, 3 to 4 cm in diameter, and irregular with shaggy edges that were undermined. The base appeared to be finely granular and pink to reddish in appearance. Indeed, from a clinical viewpoint, the ulcers could be confused with lesions due to Crohn's disease or ulcerative colitis. The appearance in my opinion was more like the ulcerations seen following long-standing ulcerative colitis with malnutrition. The determination of whether or not the condition is tuberculosis is based on a history of tuberculosis elsewhere in the body and the usual specific tests for tuberculosis, including guinea pig inoculation.

TREATMENT

Treatment must be first directed to the general disease. When that is under control, specific treatment for the ulceration at the anorectal area should be conservative and perhaps limited to distal drainage by removal of some of the shaggy edges of the ulcer to encourage healing.

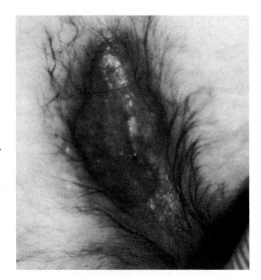

Figure 9–7. Tuberculosis.

VENEREAL DISEASE

INTRODUCTION

By definition, venereal disease is disease transmitted by sexual contact. Such disease has been seen more frequently in recent years, assuming almost epidemic proportions. This section will consider the diagnosis and treatment of several venereal diseases that occur in the anorectal area. While it is perhaps unfair to include the common wart known as condyloma acuminatum in this category, since it does not have the serious connotations of other sexually transmitted diseases, its primary mode of transmission is venereal.

Condyloma Acuminatum

These warts are irregular-shaped sessile or pedunculated structures attached to the superficial skin. The color of the lesions may be grayish pink and generally assumes the color of the surrounding skin. They may appear in clusters (Fig. 9–8), and their size varies from small excrescences of a few millimeters in diameter to a massive, cauliflower-like formation (Fig. 9–9). The disease is believed to be caused by a filterable virus, and attempts are being made to isolate the specific virus in order to make an autogenous vaccine for treatment and prevention.

PATHOLOGY

Condylomata acuminata have a distinct histologic appearance that is easily distinguishable from that of a squamous cell cancer.

DIAGNOSIS

The diagnosis would not be difficult if a reliable history could be obtained in every case. However, the appearance of these foul-smelling warts of all sizes is pathognomonic. The warts are multicentric and tend to be pedunculated. They may occur anywhere in the perianal area, anal canal, and lower

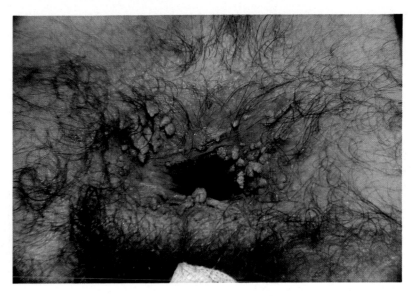

Figure 9–8. Condyloma acuminata.

rectum, and on the genitalia. It is particularly important to rule out any associated serious venereal disease.

The condyloma latum (see Fig. 9–10), which is a secondary manifestation of syphilis, is also a contagious, moist, foul-smelling wart-like lesion that may occur in the perianal area, but it is much smoother and does not raise above the skin more than a centimeter or so. The presence of a condyloma latum should immediately alert the clinician to the possibility of syphilis.

It is conceivable that a squamous cell carcinoma might be confused with these conditions. A biopsy is necessary to confirm diagnosis, although a

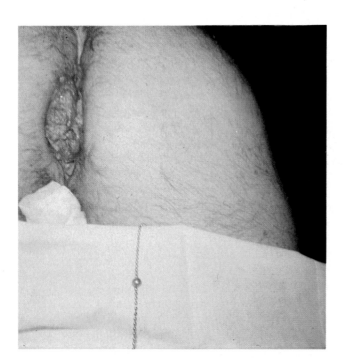

Figure 9–9. Giant-size condyloma acuminatum.

darkfield examination for *Treponema pallidum* should be performed first to rule out syphilis.

TREATMENT

Treatment of condyloma acuminatum is dependent on size, number, and the extent to which these warts involve the dentate line, crypts, and even the lower portion of the rectum. They seldom extend higher than a few centimeters above the dentate line. Small or relatively small discrete lesions that are limited to the perianal area and the lower anal canal are treated by topical application of 25 per cent podophyllin in tincture of benzoin. The physician must apply this at weekly intervals until the warts disappear. Each wart is literally soaked by this solution and the excess immediately removed with cotton. When weekly visits to the office are impossible, I have instructed a responsible member of the family—preferably a nurse—to make these applications. Topical bichloracetic acid can be used in a similar manner. The use of this agent was first proposed by Swerdlow and Salvati. The solution is applied with a sharp wood applicator and as it takes effect, the wart becomes white and frosty in appearance. Both these medications have the potential for causing serious, painful dermatitis when applications are performed in a haphazard manner. It is thus important to apply the solution with care to avoid contaminating the surrounding normal skin.

It is possible to eradicate even large clusters of warts by the persistent use of podophyllin. However, large massive wart formation, especially when it extends above the dentate line, requires surgical management under local anesthesia. All warts at the skin level are excised using a sharp scissors, with light fulguration of the base to control bleeding. Since these warts have a special predilection for the anal crypts, I usually perform excision of the crypts or at least a cryptotomy at the time of surgery to help prevent recurrence. Since these warts never grow on scar tissue, cryptotomy usually suffices.

Perhaps the most common method of treatment for more extensive warts is a combination of surgical excision and electrocoagulation using an ordinary needle-point Hyfrecator. These warts are attached to the outer layer of the superficial skin and can easily be excised and the base lightly fulgurated to prevent bleeding. Local anesthesia is used whether this is performed in the office or the hospital. These warts are autoinoculable and tend to recur. The patient should be followed very carefully in the office for at least three months after definitive surgery. The patient should be instructed carefully regarding anal hygiene and cautioned to avoid sexual contact with others who might have the warts. Laser beam is now being used and possibly may supplant electrocoagulation.

Abcarian and Sharon and others have reported excellent results with the use of autogenous vaccine in the prevention of recurrence. Some patients will refuse surgery and even local anesthesia. I have treated many such patients in the office with persistent application of the before-mentioned agents on the perianal, anal, and lower rectal areas. This method is painful and inconvenient, but if the patient is willing to make the proper number of visits to the office, the warts will eventually disappear. This type of treatment is obviously not indicated for the giant condyloma acuminatum or massive tumor-like formation. In fact, Friedberg has reported a case of squamous cell carcinoma occurring in a patient with massive warts. While malignant changes are rare, they can happen.

Syphilis

Syphilis is a contagious venereal disease that can involve any area or organ of the body. Syphilis of the anorectal area is usually acquired by rectal intercourse, although children and other innocent individuals can acquire the disease by associating with infected individuals. The infection organism is *Treponema pallidum*.

PATHOLOGY

If untreated, syphilis progresses from the chancre at the anorectal area, which is a painful, circular, indurated ulcer called the primary lesion. It is here where the organisms gain access to the tissues. Sometimes the chancre is surrounded with induration and inflammatory reaction in the lower rectum, and the inguinal lymph nodes may be enlarged. The incubation period may be anywhere from three to four weeks or even as long as three months. Multiple chancres may occur because the lesion is autoinoculable. The primary lesion or chancre is transient and heals in about six weeks. The secondary stage of syphilis is characterized by a maculopapular rash and condyloma lata. These wart-like patches appear as pink or purplish velvet-like lesions and may be multiple (Fig. 9–10). It is at this stage that syphilis is most infectious. The late or tertiary stage of syphilis may mimic almost any disease of the anorectal area and its symptoms include stricture and tumor-like formations called gummas. The late phase of syphilis can also lead to anal incontinence and the neurologic manifestations of syphilis.

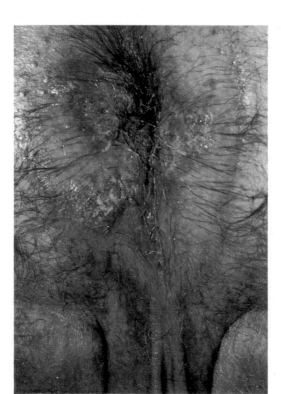

Figure 9–10. Condyloma lata.

DIAGNOSIS

Secretions from the primary lesion or ulcer (chancre) can be examined using darkfield examination for the presence of *T. pallidum*. Blood serology is not usually positive until several weeks after the chancre has disappeared.

The *differential diagnosis* is aided by the history. Anal fissure is very painful at the anus and is only unfrequently multiple. The condyloma acuminatum, a type of wart, has already been described. Lymphogranuloma venereum will be discussed separately. Chancroids are ruled out by bacterial cultures demonstrating *Hemophilus ducreyi*. The tertiary stage in which the gumma is seen is very rarely encountered at the present time. Although rare, a gumma could be confused with a tumor. Biopsy and bacteriologic studies are required to confirm the diagnosis.

TREATMENT

The drug of choice for treatment of syphilis is 2.4 million units of benzathine penicillin G in one intramuscular injection. Tetracycline or erythromycin can be given to patients who are allergic to penicillin.

Gonorrhea

Gonorrhea of the anorectal area is a contagious disease that is generally venereal in origin and involves the genitourinary tract and rectum. The infection is transmitted by direct contact, such as rectal intercourse. Children may acquire it through contaminated thermometers and enema tips.

DIAGNOSIS AND TREATMENT

Hyperemia and edema of the lower rectal mucosa with a discharge of cream-like pus from several crypts and a history of exposure is almost pathognomonic. The Gram stain may not always be positive, and special cultures are usually needed. The main point is to get a fresh specimen of the pus to the laboratory for culture and, if positive, begin treatment. Penicillin is the drug of choice in treatment.

Lymphogranuloma Venereum

Lymphogramuloma venereum is a venereal disease that is rarely seen and is characterized by phlegmonous swelling of the rectal and perineal structures, and possibly multiple fistulas. Rectal stricture is very common, especially in women.

PATHOLOGY

The virus gains access to the lymphatic system of the body by way of the external genitalia or rectum. This disease can be divided into three stages. The first stage consists of proctitis that is nonspecific in appearance. The second stage is characterized by edema, swelling in the perirectal structures, and fistulas. There may be inflammation and eventually abscess formation in

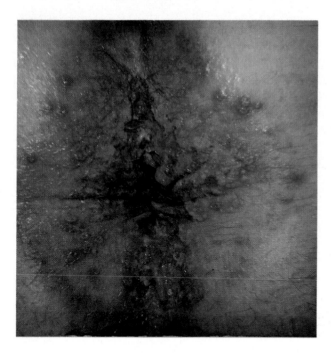

Figure 9–11. Herpes simplex.

the inguinal nodes. The late stage consists of stricture in the lower part of the rectum.

DIAGNOSIS AND TREATMENT

Diagnosis depends on the stage at which lymphogranuloma venereum is seen. Usually it is observed during the second stage and has a distinct appearance known as elephantiasis of the anogenital structures. The Frei test and the complement fixation test are specific. Syphilis is the only disease to be differentiated by darkfield examination or serology.

Tetracycline is the drug of choice. Treatment must be continued over a prolonged period of time. If the stricture causes obstruction, colostomy may eventually be necessary.

Herpes Simplex

Herpes simplex is another viral venereal disease associated with vesicles and shallow ulcers in the perianal area (Fig. 9–11). Various palliative topical applications have been described. There is no specific treatment.

REFERENCES

Abcarian, H., and Sharon, N., The effectiveness of immunotherapy in the treatment of anal condyloma acuminatum. J. Surg. Res., 22:231, 1977.

Buie, L. A., Practical Proctology. W. B. Saunders Company, Philadelphia, 1938, p. 245.

Friedberg, M. J., and Serlin, O., Condyloma acuminatum: its association with malignancy. Dis. Colon Rectum, 6:352–356, 1963.

Jackman, R. J., and McQuarrie, H. B., Hidradenitis suppurativa: its confusion with pilonidal disease and anal fistula. Am. J. Surg., 77:349, 1949.

Swerdlow, D. B., and Salvati, E. P., Condyloma acuminatum. Dis. Colon Rectum, 14:226, 1971.

CHAPTER 10

PILONIDAL DISEASE

INTRODUCTION

The term pilonidal is derived from the Latin words *pilus* and *nidus*, meaning "nest of hair." Pilonidal disease is very common in young people, the average age of occurrence being 21 years. The term cyst is not sufficiently comprehensive to describe this condition. It may present either as a sinus or group of sinuses (Fig. 10–1), as a simple lump or "cyst," or frequently as an abscess. Often a tuft of hair can be seen protruding from the opening of the cyst or sinus. The patient is often but not always a hairy individual.

Controversy persists as to whether this condition is congenital in origin or acquired. I favor the congenital theory because small sinuses over the sacrococcygeal area are present in practically every case of pilonidal disease that I have seen (Fig. 10–2A). These sinuses may be so small that a lachrymal probe cannot be made to pass their orifices but they can be seen (Fig. 10–3). At operation, I have noticed that while the entrances of these sinuses are lined by normal epithelium, the cyst or abscess cavity is lined by granulation tissue. Spencer has been able to demonstrate the presence of hair follicles in the lining of the cyst itself.

The congenital theory, however, does not explain the absence of sinuses in the newborn or the occasional pilonidal cysts that develop between a barber's fingers; neither does it explain the reason for recurrence of pilonidal cysts. These patients are referred to the proctologist because of the frequent confusion between this disease and anal fistula.

DIAGNOSIS

The key words in dealing with pilonidal disease are hair and infection. The practitioner dealing with pilonidal disease must realize that the infection occurs in an area confined by skin posteriorly and by the fascia of the sacrum anteriorly. There are no lateral limits to the space, and therefore it is not a space in the usual sense of the word, though we might designate this the pilonidal or retrosacral space. A pilonidal cyst should not be confused with the easily recognizable pilonidal dimple (Fig. 10–2B). These dimples occur in the midline near the tip of the coccyx and are formed by traction on the skin

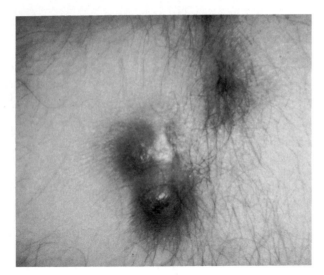

Figure 10–1. Pilonidal disease.

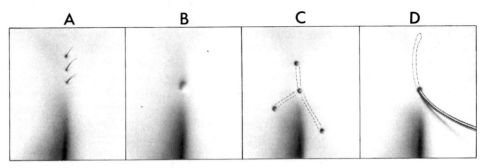

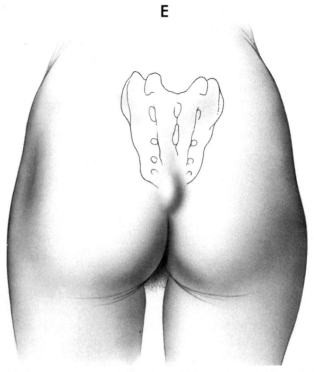

Figure 10–2. Pilonidal disease. *A,* Multiple sinuses with shafts of hair protruding from the orifices. *B,* Harmless pilonidal dimple. *C,* Multiple sinuses. *D,* Probe passed into a sinus tract. **E,** Pilonidal abscess.

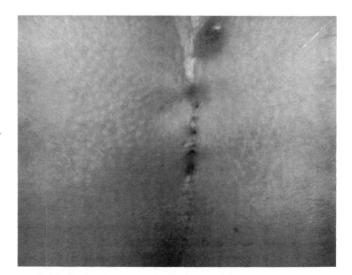

Figure 10–3. Pilonidal disease showing tiny sinuses in midline.

by fibrous bands that are inserted in the coccyx. The pilonidal dimple is normal and should not be excised. It is not a sinus and is lined by normal epithelium. I have seen this normal structure frequently in infants, and, while harmless, it often is of major concern to the mother. Although I advise against excision of the pilonidal dimple, some mothers will insist on having it removed.

True pilonidal disease usually presents as an abscess on or close to the midline over the sacrococcygeal area (Fig. 10–4). There may be a history of recurrent abscesses. Sometimes, the infection is merely smoldering and the patient has a painful nodule, possibly recurrent with periods of remission over months or even years. I have seen many patients in which the infection never develops into a true abscess. Frequently, the patient notes only moisture and irritation of the skin over the sacrococcygeal area and this exudate may have an objectionable odor.

Careful examination with excellent lighting may reveal one or more sinuses in the exact midline (Fig. 10–2C). Pilonidal disease is seldom present without at least one of these sinuses. The entrance to these sinuses is a continuation of normal skin. A shaft or tuft of hair often protrudes from the

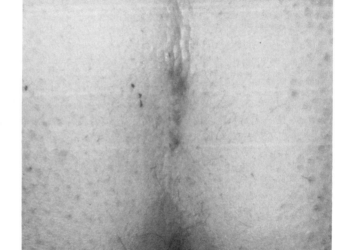

Figure 10–4. Pilonidal abscess.

opening or openings, but not in every case. Pus or watery fluid in tiny amounts may exude from these openings. The surrounding skin may be hyperemic from irritation.

Wide-mouthed sinuses are a manifestation of advanced disease after at least one abscess has formed. Such sinuses are not limited to the midline but can be found anywhere on the sacrococcygeal area, the buttocks, or even the perineum anterior to the anus. They are mere extensions of the same disease and are connected with one another by tracts. Whenever one suspects a pilonidal cyst, a careful history, inspection, palpation, probing (Fig. 10–2D) or instrumentation, and, when necessary, proper laboratory tests, are indicated.

When a patient experiences pain and swelling, the infection may have become a huge abscess, which may be associated with fever (Figs. 10–2E and 10–5A). If the patient complains of pain without swelling, the abscess may be deep and next to the fascia of the sacrum (Fig. 10–5B). Even careful palpation may not reveal it, especially when the patient is obese. In other words, the infection can be severe or mild. One must remember that this disease is common in very young people. The pain is not a product of their imagination. If the physician relates the above-mentioned symptoms to a practical knowledge of anatomy and pathology, management of these problems will proceed quite simply and skillfully.

On rare occasions, a patient may present with a painless, round or elliptical soft mass from 1 to 3 cm in diameter over the sacrococcygeal area. This is a true cyst with a definite wall and hair on the inside.

The *differential diagnosis* is usually not difficult. Furuncle, anal fistula, and hidradenitis suppurativa are the common diseases that may be confused with pilonidal disease. As long as one realizes that pilonidal disease originates as sinuses in the midline that may from there extend elsewhere, differential diagnosis should not pose a problem.

Anal fistula can be ruled out by the fact that the induration does not enter the anal canal and that there is no evidence of a primary opening or fistula originating in a diseased crypt. Although a pilonidal cyst may extend very close to the anus and indeed may extend anterior to the anus on the perineum, skillful palpation can very readily confirm the diagnosis.

Sinuses from imbedded foreign bodies, congenital deformities, teratomas, or actinomycosis are rare possibilities in diagnosis. Spina bifida and sacrococcygeal teratomata are so dramatic in their appearance that they do not pose a problem in the differential diagnosis.

TREATMENT

The treatment for pilonidal disease is relatively simple but requires proper judgment and timing. The form of management used depends on the stage at which the disease presents. Not all patients suffering from pilonidal disease want to or should be treated surgically. If one sees a shallow sinus with a tuft of hair protruding from it and that cannot be probed farther than 1 to 1½ inches in the subcutaneous tissue, conservative management might be tried, although the patient should be told that development of an abscess is always a possibility. Conservative management requires scrupulous cleansing of the area and the application of phenol utilizing a small probe. The phenol works by destroying the epithelial lining in the tract and producing a temporary inflammatory reaction and consequent healing. I have followed a

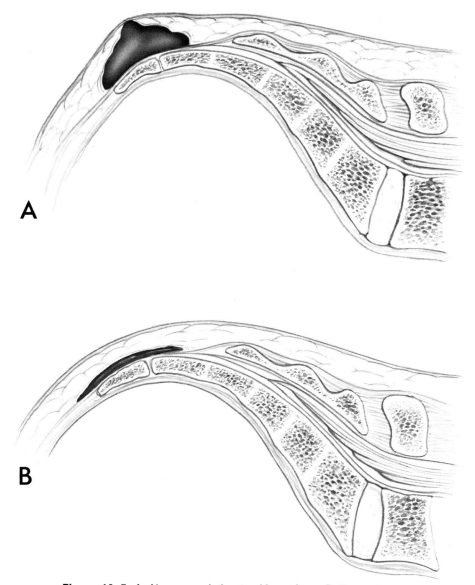

Figure 10–5. *A*, Abscess pointing to skin surface. *B*, Deep abscess.

number of patients for many years who did not want either surgery or phenol applications. Daily cleansing of the area with cotton soaked in witch hazel was advised. These patients are all of the very hairy type and generally obese. At the present time they are doing well and without complications.

In the presence of an abscess, it is usually safest to incise and drain immediately under local anesthesia. While general anesthesia may be considered for extensive pilonidal disease with acute cellulitis and fever and other systemic symptoms, I have exclusively used local anesthesia for pilonidal disease since 1954. The local anesthetic is infiltrated intradermally along the course of the proposed incision, which is determined by the size of the abscess (Figs. 10–6 and 10–7A). The incision should be almost as long as the abscess (Fig. 10–7B). The entire cyst cavity can be exposed and the skin trimmed after careful probing to avoid overlooking extensions of the cyst. These can be treated similarly. If in doubt, drain only. One should be careful not to

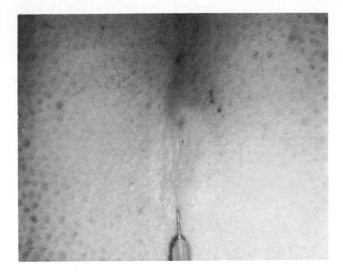

Figure 10–6. Intradermal infiltration of anesthetic agent.

create a false passage; it is easy to push a probe through the normal subcutaneous tissue. It is important to recognize necrotic inflammatory granulating tissue as the incision is made in the skin. This, correlated with the findings of the probing, should determine the extent of the incisions. Adequate drainage is imperative (Fig. 10–8). Routine bacterial cultures are taken and Oxycel gauze is placed in the cavity to encourage hemostasis of the wound edges and to keep the skin incision open for drainage. Pressure

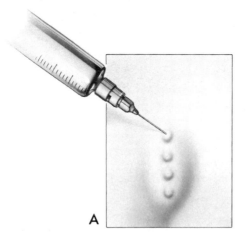

A

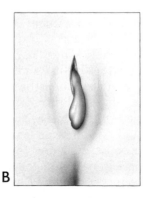

B

Figure 10–7. *A,* Anesthetic agent injected intradermally. *B,* Incision has been made. Pus is exuding.

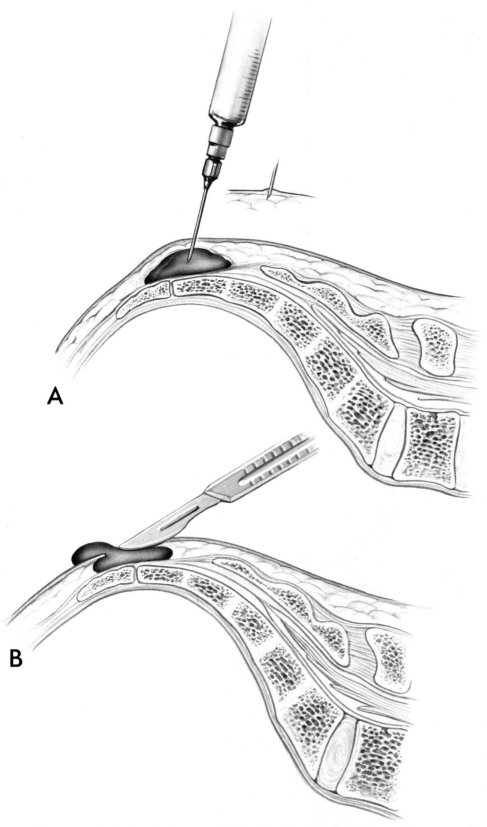

Figure 10–8. *A,* Anesthetic agent injected intradermally and then subcutaneously prior to diagnostic tap of deep abscess. *B,* Incision and drainage of deep abscess.

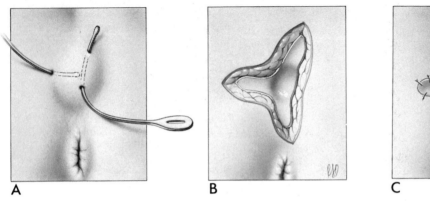

Figure 10–9. *A,* Probes in multiple tracts. *B,* All tracts opened by incising the anesthetized skin overlying the probes. *C,* Suturing the skin to the posterior wall of the tract.

gauze dressings are placed by strapping the buttocks with adhesive. The patient may go home immediately from the office. Dressings are removed the following day and sitz baths begun.

For smaller abscess, the surgery is completed in one stage. For large abscesses, those over 4 inches in diameter, surgery for pilonidal disease becomes a staged operation, with immediate incision and drainage of the lesion, followed by incision of subsidiary tracts after inflammation has subsided.

I believe that incision of all tracts and trimming of the skin edges under local anesthesia are all that is necessary to cure pilonidal disease (Fig. 10–9*A* and *B*). I have operated on many patients, including my own, for recurrence following primary closure (Fig. 10–10). It is entirely unnecessary to excise the area of pilonidal disease down to the fascia of the sacrum. This is radical surgery that produces a nasty scar and abnormal anatomic relationships. Marsupialization is an excellent procedure (Figs. 10–9*C* and 10–11). The intent of marsupialization is to incise all of the tracts leaving the posterior wall of the sinuses intact. The granulation tissue may be removed with dry

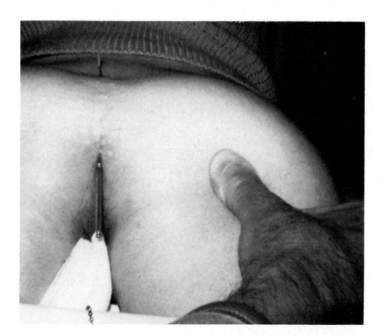

Figure 10–10. Recurrent disease after primary closure.

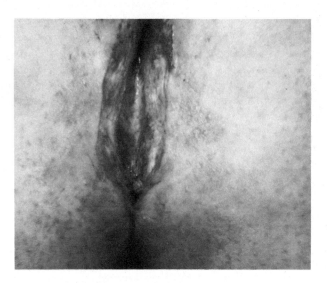

Figure 10–11. Technic of marsupialization.

gauze in an effort to find any subsidiary tracts. The probe is helpful at this point. If feasible, the skin can then be sewed to the edge of the posterior wall of the tracts using interrupted or continuous lock-stitch sutures of triple 0 chromic catgut. If it is not feasible to marsupialize with suture, after trimming the skin, a needle-point Hyfrecator may be used to lightly fulgurate the skin to avoid bleeding. I do not hesitate to fulgurate all potential bleeding areas thoroughly because many of these patients live quite a distance from the office and bleeding must be prevented.

Since these patients are operated on in the office, no preoperative sedation is given. I find that patients suffer more from medication given preoperatively than they do from the local anesthetic agent. The local anesthetic used is 0.5 per cent lidocaine with epinephrine 1:200,000. After strapping the buttocks apart and shaving the area, as well as preparing it with povidone-iodine, the, local anesthetic agent is injected intradermally entirely around all the areas to be incised. Then, utilizing a longer needle, the subcutaneous tissue is infiltrated with local anesthesia right down to the fascia of the sacrum well away from the diseased area.

As stated previously, it is rare to find a well-delineated pilonidal cyst without abscess or some evidence of infection as the presenting sign. However, when it occurs a longitudinal incision over the cyst is necessary (Fig. 10–12A). In order to avoid breaking into the cyst, the skin that appears to be adherent is excised along with the cyst. These cysts are easily "peeled" out and off the fascia of the sacrum. One is inclined to close the wounds and allow for primary healing. However, they heal just as quickly if the redundant surrounding skin is removed (Fig. 10–12B), hemostasis of the wound edges obtained by the use of the Hyfrecator, and Oxycel gauze placed in the cavity. A pressure dressing (Fig. 10–13) is applied for one or two days, strapping the buttocks with adhesive tape to produce the desired result. The dressings are then removed, and only cotton, kept in place by snugly fitting underwear, is used to absorb any drainage from the wound. Medication for pain is usually required for one or two days.

Operations on large abscesses may keep a patient away from school or a desk job for a day or two. Those whose job entails heavy manual work should stay at home for one or two weeks. Depending on the circumstances, patients with small abscesses or small pilonidal cysts treated in the office may go back

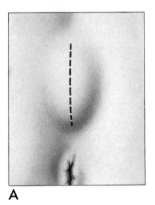

A

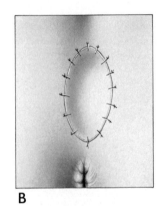

B

Figure 10–12. A, Incision of skin overlying a true cyst. B, Skin sutured to edges of fascia after the cyst has been "peeled" out.

Figure 10–13. A, Pressure dressing that is used in all patients. B, Cross-section of pressure dressing.

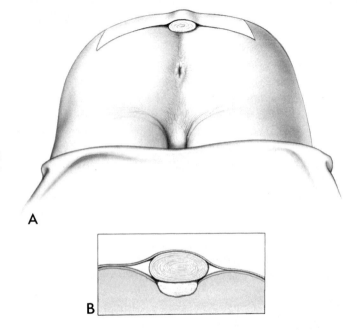

A

B

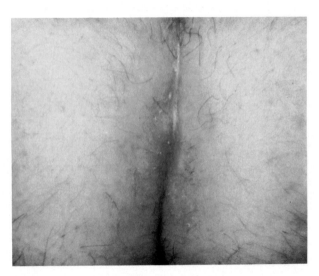

Figure 10–14. Healed wound.

to work the following day; however, they must report for postoperative care every week until healing is complete.

POSTOPERATIVE CARE

After removal of the dressings, postoperative care is begun. Cleanliness is the key word in postoperative care. The wounds should be kept apart to avoid the so-called bridging effect. Sitz baths certainly make the patient more comfortable and should be utilized if feasible. The big problem in postoperative care is keeping the hair immediately around the wound shaved. A razor may be used and at times a sharp scissors with a forceps. After two weeks, if granulation becomes a problem, it can be curretted as needed. Most wounds are completely healed in four to six weeks (Fig. 10–14). Those patients having only incision and drainage of the abscess may often have complete incision of the subsidiary tracts within one week.

Some patients (2 per cent), chiefly obese patients, take longer to heal. However, this does not keep them from going back to work, although it does require that they return to the doctor's office for follow-up visits for an indefinite period of time. After several months of poor healing and depending upon the reaction of the patient, I excise any unhealed wounds completely. In other words, trimming of the skin is not enough in these cases; they also require total excision of the infected posterior wall of the tracts or cysts.

SUMMARY

Small sinuses can sometimes be eradicated by simple cleanliness and occasional application of phenol to the tract. However, a cyst of any size requires either complete excision, incision and drainage, marsupialization, or occasionally primary closure. On rare occasions when the cyst has a definite wall that shells out very easily without spillage, the wound may be closed. However, primary closure in the presence of infection or when the cyst does not have a definite cyst wall is usually followed by recurrence of the disease. The great majority of patients suffering from pilonidal disease are infected and they should be treated accordingly. Usually all that is necessary is incision and trimming of the skin edges. It is unnecessary to attempt to excise all infected tissue down to the fascia of the sacrum. Some surgeons, in an effort to close large wounds following excision of the cyst, will try vainly to use relaxing incisions on the buttocks, swinging over large flaps of skin and fat and even the gluteal muscle to close the defect. I would advise the use of the simple marsupialization method first, and if this fails, complete excision down to the fascia can be performed.

REFERENCES

Seebrechts, P., Personal communication, 1984.
Spencer, R., Personal communication, 1970.

11 CHAPTER

CROHN'S DISEASE

INTRODUCTION

Crohn's disease is evolving as the most common and completely perplexing segment of inflammatory bowel disease. Sophisticated approaches to disease generally cannot be applied to Crohn's disease, because there is no hard information available concerning its etiology and treatment. Crohn's disease may involve any area of the alimentary canal from the mouth to the anus. The disease is characterized by "skip areas," anal fistulas, and a tendency to recur after both medical and surgical treatment. It is unpredictable in its manifestations in the gastrointestinal tract as well as in its systemic complications. These complications can be severe and difficult to treat because of the varying amounts of small bowel involvement, and often result in serious if not insurmountable nutritional problems. Most clinicians consider the disease to be incurable.

Chronic ulcerative colitis, the other large segment of inflammatory bowel disease, is considered to be curable. Although this disease may also be associated with systemic complications, the internal manifestations are limited to the colon and rectum. A cure requires colectomy and ileostomy, although efforts are now being made to eliminate the need for ileostomy. Fortunately, most of these patients can be controlled medically. I emphasize the word control, since we cannot consider patients maintained on a medical regimen to be cured.

For teaching purposes, and more specifically to serve the purposes of this book, the two major types of inflammatory bowel disease will be discussed individually. However, the reader should remember the striking similarities between these conditions and the dearth of essential or concrete information concerning either of them. Crohn's disease is relatively and historically a new disease. Most institutions have not, and perhaps cannot, reclassify and thus separate it from ulcerative colitis. It is apparent that lack of a proper classification system makes the task of advancing knowledge of this disease very difficult.

This chapter will summarize what little is known of Crohn's disease from the literature and, where appropriate, my own experience.

ETIOLOGY

The exact etiology of Crohn's disease is unknown. That more than 100 local and systemic complications have been described and that virtually all organ systems may be involved might indicate that it is a general disease of multicentric origin. It originates most frequently in the distal ileum, and this fact alone suggests that this area of the intestinal tract may play a role in etiology.

PATHOLOGY

Crohn's disease (transmural proctocolitis, regional enteritis) involves all layers of the bowel. Because the disease involves the wall of the bowel and its mesentery more heavily than the mucosa, bleeding is not an outstanding feature of this disease. It is a chronic granulomatous process that causes thickening of both the wall of the bowel and its mesentery. The glands in the mesentery are thickened and tend to be confluent with one another, forming abscesses and fistulas of all types, with areas of normal bowel, or "skip areas," in between.

The abnormal bowel is characterized by "fat wrapping" and punctate areas on the serosa, creating a salt-and-pepper appearance. The fat wrapping is nature's way of sealing off minute abscesses. The exact distribution of these lesions in the intestinal tract is unknown because the disease may be present without gross evidence of involvement. Approximately 50 per cent of these lesions involve the ileum; 20 per cent, the colon; and 10 to 20 per cent, the anorectal area. However, there are many unusual combinations and this distribution should be regarded as a rough guide only (Fig. 11–1).

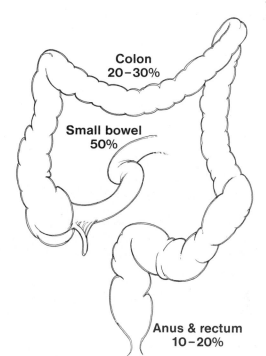

Figure 11–1. Distribution of Crohn's disease in colon and rectum.

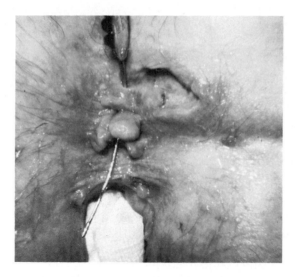

Figure 11–2. Anorectal ulcerations and fistula in Crohn's disease.

The lesions have a tendency to produce long stenotic areas in the bowel and lacunar-like abscesses just beneath the serosa. However, abscesses may occur anywhere in the wall of the bowel and mesentery. The mucosa may have a cobblestone appearance, and there may be long slit-like secondary ulcers.

Anorectal Crohn's disease is characterized by large, shaggy ulcerations with undermined skin edges, bizarre fistulas, thickening of the tissues, and a tendency to stenosis of the anorectal area (Figs. 11–2 and 11–3). It may be associated with similar disease higher in the intestinal tract, or it may precede by many years development of gross disease elsewhere.

Toxic megacolon as well as dilation of the ileum may occur, as they do in ulcerative colitis, although to a lesser degree. Cancer is also less common in the colon involved by Crohn's disease, the incidence of cancer being approximately half that found in conjunction with ulcerative colitis. There are approximately 50 cases of small bowel cancer reported in the literature. Perforation and obstruction, however, are more common in Crohn's disease than in ulcerative colitis.

Recurrence is the distinctive feature of this disease. The literature indicates a recurrence rate of 40 to 60 per cent. These rates are directly

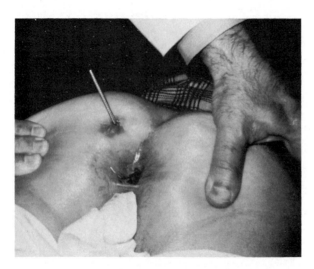

Figure 11–3. Fistula in Crohn's disease.

related to the length of follow-up. Glotzer et al. report a recurrence rate of zero per cent following proctocolectomy with ileostomy. Their patients were followed from 1 to 8 years. Korelitz et al. report a recurrence rate of 40 per cent following proctolectomy with ileostomy. Their patients were followed from 1 to 30 years.

In evaluating recurrence rates it is important to realize that in 20 per cent of patients it is impossible to differentiate ulcerative colitis from Crohn's disease. Furthermore, some patients with ileostomy and proctocolectomy may develop a form of ileitis due to functional problems of the ileostomy rather than to actual Crohn's disease. Weakley states that in Crohn's disease limited to the colon and rectum, proctocolectomy resulted in a recurrence rate approaching zero.

Dysplasia in chronic ulcerative colitis detected by histologic examination of specimens taken at biopsy from relatively normal mucosa will certainly help to detect those colons apt to develop cancer. The hyperchromatic nuclei and other histologic features are not difficult to recognize. At our present state of knowledge concerning dysplasia, it is desirable to take biopsy specimens from various areas of the colon. Jagelman and Veidenheimer claim that specimens taken through the regular rigid sigmoidoscope may eventually prove sufficient to make the diagnosis. In fact, in cooperation with the World Health Organization, Morson is preparing slides to be distributed to all pathologists, thereby making it possible for this diagnosis to be made anywhere in the world.

DIAGNOSIS

When this unpredictable disease is suspected, an unusual effort must be made to make a complete diagnosis. Nothing must be overlooked or neglected. The history and physical are especially important, since the disease may present as appendicitis or any one of many clinical manifestations. Stool examinations are essential to rule out specific bacterial, parasitic, or fungal infections. Comprehensive blood tests, a chest x-ray, a flat plate of the abdomen, and upper and lower GI series including CT scans are essential. Complete endoscopic investigation, including colonoscopy, is also important. Mucosal biopsy, including histologic examination of the bizarre anorectal lesions, when these are present, is insufficient, since granulomas are present in only 50 per cent of tissue taken at random biopsy (Fig. 11–4).

HISTORY AND PHYSICAL EXAMINATION

The findings depend on the stage of the disease and the area involved. Crohn's disease may present simply as ileitis with episodes of fever, diarrhea, and abdominal pain limited to the right lower quadrant. Bleeding is seldom a feature. It may present as acute appendicitis, as a ruptured appendix, or as obstruction. Sometimes only a mass is found on palpation, usually in the right lower quadrant, although such a mass may be found anywhere in the abdomen. Those presenting with abscesses may exhibit them anywhere in the abdomen or elsewhere.

Malnutrition with loss of weight, secondary ulcers in the mouth (Fig. 11–5), and infections of the skin as well as intestinal signs including cutaneous fistula may occasionally be the presenting problem in extensive and neglected disease.

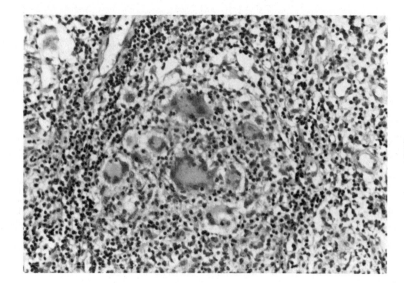

Figure 11–4. Photomicrograph from biopsy of anorectal Crohn's disease.

INSTRUMENTATION

On endoscopic examination, Crohn's disease of the rectum and colon will display the typical cobblestone appearance with shaggy, slit-like ulcers (Fig. 11–6). Skip areas are revealed by areas or segments of normal bowel. When the entire colon and even the distal ileum is examined by the colonoscope, a similar appearance will be noted. Areas of stenosis may prevent complete examination by a colonoscope of the usual diameter, and a pediatric colonoscope or duodenoscope may be necessary.

Surprisingly, the proctosigmoidsocopic examination may be essentially negative except for a few nonspecific superficial hyperemic ulcers at the rectosigmoid junction. These may be due to a loop of ileum, involved by ileitis, lying in the pelvis and in close proximity to the rectosigmoid. While this finding does not necessarily mean that this part of the colon is involved by Crohn's disease, it suggests the necessity for further study. On the other hand, the colon in this area may be involved with Crohn's disease, and an enterocolic fistula may be present.

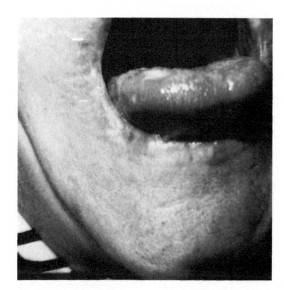

Figure 11–5. Secondary ulcers of mouth in Crohn's disease.

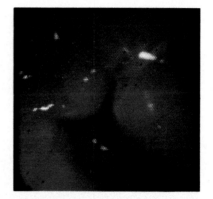

Figure 11–6. Endoscopic appearance of Crohn's disease.

RADIOLOGIC EXAMINATION

Inflammatory disease of the gastrointestinal tract makes radiologic examinations mandatory. In patients with suspected obstruction and/or perforation with or without abscess and/or fistula formation, the flat plate of the abdomen is mandatory. When occult abscesses are suspected, CT scan and ultrasound examination may also be indicated. Although free air from perforation into the general peritoneal cavity is seldom encountered, the use of barium enema in suspected complicated cases should be used with caution. Barium and feces in the general peritoneal cavity can be a lethal combination. In such cases, an aqueous solution of hypopaque material (Gastrografin) may be of help in demonstrating perforations with abscesses and fistulas. The average patient seen in the office does not have these complications, and the use of double-contrast studies with barium is feasible.

Marshak and other radiologists having vast experience with inflammatory bowel disease have described the pathognomonic radiologic signs. These include cobblestone appearance, lacunar subserosal longitudinal abscesses, and skip areas in the colon by barium enema (Fig. 11–7), and in the small bowel by barium meal. Long, narrow stenotic areas allow only a trickle of barium to pass through to produce the "string" sign when visualized radiographically. These radiologists were able to differentiate ulcerative colitis from Crohn's disease in practically all subjects, the only exception being that very small percentage of patients in whom elements of both diseases coexist.

Differential Diagnosis

Appendicitis, tuberculosis, ulcerative colitis, ischemic colitis due to vascular insufficiency, the colitis which occurs proximal to obstructions due to cancer, and other specific colitides are among the entities to be differentiated.

TREATMENT

The belief that ulcerative colitis can be cured by surgery and that Crohn's disease cannot be cured by surgery is gradually losing validity except in cases involving the small bowel. Certainly in early cases without complications, medical management seems logical. Even without treatment uncomplicated Crohn's disease can run an indefinite course almost to a point of burning itself out before the onset of complications.

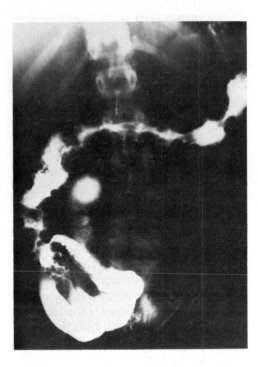

Figure 11–7. Colon x-ray in Crohn's disease.

Accurate diagnosis, especially as to the area(s) of the gastrointestinal tract involved and the degree of obstruction and complications present, is crucial in treatment. For example, when there is impending obstruction it is unwise to persist in use of a high-residue diet.

Surgical Management

Because of the great tendency of recurrence, surgery is delayed as long as possible. Of course, obstruction, toxic megacolon, perforation with abscess and fistula formation, as well as intractability may make surgery mandatory.

Although surgery may not be curative, it could well be life-saving. To serve the purpose of this book, only the most frequent operations performed for Crohn's disease will be listed. In order of frequency, based on my experience, the following operations are employed: incision and drainage of perirectal abscesses, anal fistulectomy, proctolectomy with permanent ileostomy, right colon resection, resection of portions of the small bowel, and entero-enterostomy or other forms of bypass procedures.

Medical Management

Although there is no specific medical treatment, it is possible to "buy time" with the use of a modified low-residue diet, sulfasalazine (Azulfidine), and steroids. This treatment is used only when the greater part of the small bowel and colon is involved without complications.

Sulfasalazine (Azulfidine). Sulfasalazine is a combination of sulfa and salicylic acid introduced from Sweden to the United States by Bargen. The "azo-" linkage makes it possible for the combined drug to get to the colon in larger amounts than if either compound were used alone. Most of it is metabolized. It is not superior to steroids and its mode of action is not known.

Sulfasalazine should be reserved for patients with mild to moderately severe disease. Side effects occur in over 35 per cent of patients with prolonged use in dosages of over 1.5 to 2 gm daily. Side effects include nausea, headache, anorexia, abdominal pain, myalgia, arthralgia, fever, drug rash, and hematologic side effects such as agranulocytosis, leukopenia, pancytopenia, thrombocytopenia, purpura, Heinz bodies with or without anemia, and hemolytic anemia. The drug may also interfere with absorption of folic acid. Sulfasalazine may also cause peripheral neuropathy, acute pancreatitis, liver and lung disease, and possible harmful effects on pregnant patients (since it traverses the placental barrier).

I have used sulfasalazine in approximately 671 colitis patients over a period of 37 years, giving a maintenance dose of only 1 gm daily for two years after an initial dose of 4 gm daily for two to six weeks. The only side effects noted were occasional nausea and headache, which may be prevented by having the patient take the drug with milk, six cases of skin rash, and four cases of leukopenia. One patient gave birth to a deformed child while on therapy, although the connection cannot be proved.

Steroids. Well-controlled studies demonstrate the superiority of steroids over placebos. Furthermore, systemic steroids are more effective than topical steroids. Combination therapy including Azulfidine and steroids is still more effective. The response rate is proportional to the amount of steroids given. However, large doses seldom are necessary. Furthermore, side effects are directly related to size of the dosage.

Systemic steroids are reserved for patients with acute moderate to severe attacks of Crohn's disease. These patients should be treated by daily doses of 200 to 300 mg of hydrocortisone or 40 to 60 mg of prednisone unless contraindicated by hypertension, diabetes, osteoporosis, severe sepsis, or psychosis. The optimal mode of administration of oral steroids, the varied response of the individual, the diurnal cycle of endogenous secretion of steroids, or the reasons for the initial effective response are not clearly defined. However, it is important to maintain effective dosages for months or even years. Thus the physician should gradually reduce the amount to the lowest effective dose and specify divided doses. One can change from hydrocortisone to prednisone or vice versa. While steroids may have a beneficial effect on Crohn's disease, according to Shorter, they will not reduce the incidence of recurrence. Steroids do not increase the incidence of perforation of the colon.

It should be emphasized that the severely ill patient needs supportive treatment such as plasma albumin, blood, and antibiotics. Those who have been on steroids need additional intravenous steroids (ACTH or hydrocortisone). Topical steroids such as rectal drip, suppositories, and Cortenema or Cortifoam should be used to relieve tenesmus and to help generally. It must be remembered that 30 per cent or more of the steroid can be absorbed through topical administration. Since the effect of topical steroid therapy has not been completely evaluated, it is not known how much of the colon is reached by this mode of therapy.

Immunosuppressive Drugs. I have not had experience with immunosuppressive drugs. Azathioprine has proved to be the most popular of the cytotoxic drugs, which are thought to be anti-inflammatory and antiviral. Azathioprine may make it possible to reduce the amount of steroids used or eliminate them completely. Long-term administration of azathioprine may be associated with fever, skin rashes, bone marrow suppression, pancytopenia, cholestatic jaundice, and pancreatitis. Leukopenia and thrombocytopenia have occurred with 6-mercaptopurine, a major metabolite of azathioprine, as well as with large doses of azathioprine. These problems have discouraged the use of immunosuppressive therapy.

Antibiotics. The acutely ill patient should receive antibiotics, of which the most commonly used are tetracycline and ampicillin. When given to patients for conditions other than colitis, these drugs can actually produce a form of nonspecific colitis or even a specific superinfection by staphylococci or fungi. When given to the patient with Crohn's disease, tetracycline and ampicillin can aggravate the colitis, and clindomycin and gentamycin can cause membranous colitis. Cultures and sensitivity studies of the blood and stool are generally run when the use of antibiotics is under consideration. Should a pathogen be cultured from the blood or stool, the antibiotic used would be determined by the sensitivity tests.

Supportive Measures

Inflammatory bowel disease requires correction of dehydration, electrolyte disturbances, anemia, and hypoproteinemia. Shock from hemorrhage, fluid loss, or gram-negative sepsis must be treated vigorously by rapid fluid replacement, and, as needed, blood and antibiotics. Central venous manometry may be necessary in hypovolemic shock.

Depletion of sodium, chloride, and potassium may result from diarrhea and occasionally from associated vomiting. Depletion of potassium is especially apt to occur from the use of steroids with poor absorption from the disease. Calcium salts must be given intravenously, and occasionally magnesium must be given intramuscularly if it is not tolerated by mouth.

Patients with inflammatory bowel disease become anemic as a result of blood loss; poor absorption of the hematinic factors iron, folic acid, and vitamin B_{12}; a poor diet; bone marrow depression associated with the toxic illness; or hemolysis due to sulfasalazine. Dehydration often masks the degree of anemia. Transfusions may be necessary in patients with acute blood loss. Iron may be given to patients with a chronic condition, although when given orally iron may aggravate the colitis; in these cases, intramuscular iron should be used. Folic acid supplements may be given in a 1-mg oral dose each day.

Blood-clotting disturbances from hepatic disease, malabsorption of vitamin K as a result of the disease, or prolonged intake of antibiotics may require supplemental injections of vitamin K. Hypoproteinemia may be corrected by human albumin, 25 to 50 gm intravenously daily. Amino acids are not as useful for this purpose because of their rapid passage through the circulation and into the urine. Patients with hypoxia from whatever cause must have their blood gas values corrected. Patients with inflammatory bowel disease are prone to phlebitis and pulmonary embolization.

Nutritional Support

Since this is a disease of deficiencies created by poor absorption of the various food elements, special diets, intravenous nutrition, and even total parenteral hyperalimentation must be considered, depending on the severity of the disease. For instance, when fat is poorly absorbed and steatorrhea is evident, a prepared food (Portagen) that contains medium-chain triglycerides (MCT) may be given. The high osmolality of MCT may aggravate the diarrhea, however, and the amount should be limited to 100 gm daily. If cirrhosis of the liver is present, these preparations should not be given.

Depending on laboratory studies, deficiencies in iron, calcium, folic acid, vitamin B_{12} (by injection each month), sodium, potassium, bicarbonate, and zinc supplements are indicated. According to Shorter, magnesium deficiency is apt to occur in severe malabsorption problems. If magnesium deficiency exists, the patient should receive intramuscular injections of magnesium sulfate. A local anesthetic will reduce the pain of the injection.

Elemental diets containing amino acids, sugar, fats, multivitamin supplements including vitamin K, iron, magnesium, calcium, copper, zinc, and iodine are available. Vivonex and Flexical are two examples. These preparations are absorbable even if only 100 cm of functionally absorptive intestine is present. They are employed only when the patient is not able to ingest or absorb proteins and calories on a regular diet. Management of these therapeutic diets requires close monitoring with blood and urine studies to avoid further serious nutritional deficiencies. Severely ill patients require total parenteral hyperalimentation, and such treatment should be controlled by physicians skilled in its management.

REFERENCES

Glotzer, D. J., Stone, P. A., and Paterson, J. F., Prognosis after surgical treatment of granulomatous colitis. N. Engl. J. Med., 277:273, 1967.

Jagelman, D. G., and Veidenheimer, M. C., Personal communication, 1983.

Kirsner, J. B., and Shorter, R. G. (eds.), Inflammatory Bowel Disease. Lea & Febiger, Philadelphia, 1975.

Korelitz, B. I., Persent, D. H., and Alpert, L. I., et al., Recurrent regional ileitis after ileostomy and colectomy for granulomatous colitis. N. Engl. J. Med., 287:110–114, 1972.

Marshak, R. H., and Lindner, A. E., Radiologic diagnosis of chronic ulcerative colitis and Crohn's disease in the colon. *In* Kirsner, J. B., and Shorter, R. G. (eds.), Inflammatory Bowel Disease. Lea & Febiger, Philadelphia, 1975, pp. 241–276.

Morson, B. C., and Pang, L. S., Rectal biopsy as an aid to cancer control in ulcerative colitis. Gut, 8:423–434, 1967.

ULCERATIVE COLITIS

INTRODUCTION

There are no hard facts available that prove ulcerative colitis has a specific cause. In 1924, Bargen isolated a gram-positive diplostreptococcus from patients suffering from this disease; he claimed that the disease could be reproduced in experimental animals and that a prepared vaccine would benefit patients. This concept gained some popularity for several years and then was abandoned because others could not duplicate these results. While various other theories have been described, none as yet has proved universally applicable.

Ulcerative colitis is a disease of Western civilization, afflicting both sexes and usually manifesting itself in the third decade of life, although in recent years it has been found with increasing frequency in the elderly. It is more common in Jews than in non-Jews. In America, the incidence is 6 per 100,000 population.

Many believe the rectum is always involved in ulcerative colitis (a more accurate term might be proctocolitis). The disease almost always begins in the rectum, which is the area most severely involved, and then migrates relentlessly higher in the colon after a variable period of time. The exception to this rule is the 5 to 10 per cent of cases in which only a portion of the rectum is involved (Fig. 12–1). Only 10 per cent of these patients show further migration. This is really a mild proctitis, more of a nuisance than a disease. It is difficult to reassure the patient because of the intermittent discharge of bloody mucus from the rectum. For some unknown reason, the condition does not exhibit the potential for cancer and the other serious complications that are seen in ulcerative colitis or Crohn's disease.

According to the literature, in 18 per cent of cases only the rectum and rectosigmoid are involved. The rectum and left colon are involved in 28 per cent of patients, and the entire rectum and colon are involved in 36 per cent of patients. Nine per cent of cases are classified as enterocolitis. However, since only the colon and rectum are involved in ulcerative colitis, it is believed and I concur that this involvement of the distal ileum is a "backwash ileitis," which exhibits superficial edema with tiny ulcerations of the mucosa. The condition is harmless and disappears when the colitis is treated properly.

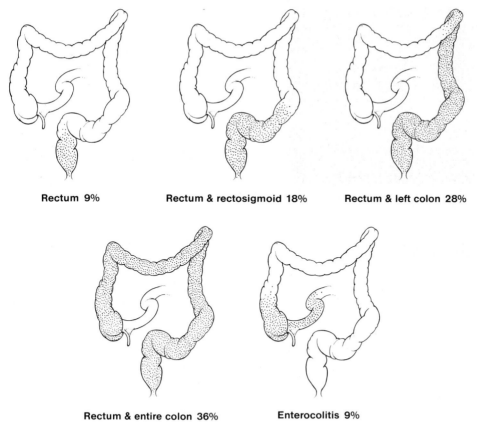

Rectum 9%   **Rectum & rectosigmoid 18%**   **Rectum & left colon 28%**

Rectum & entire colon 36%   **Enterocolitis 9%**

Figure 12–1. Distribution of ulcerative colitis in the colon.

Segmental ulcerative colitis does occur, but the ileum is not involved. Thus cases classified as ileocolitis should be carefully reviewed for Crohn's disease, which can involve any area of the alimentary canal.

PATHOLOGY

In most cases, ulcerative colitis is confined to the mucosa and submucosa. However, as gross secondary ulceration progresses, the entire wall of the bowel is involved and gradually destroyed. In fact, some portions of the colon may become thin and distended like a sausage skin. This is known as toxic megacolon and may lead to perforation. Fortunately, the majority of colitis patients are controlled either spontaneously or by treatment long before these serious manifestations develop. Some researchers have described destruction of the myenteric plexus as a cause of toxic megacolon. Others question this hypothesis.

The pathognomonic sign is that the disease at an early stage is limited to the mucosa and easily missed by palpation (Fig. 12–2). Later the colon is thickened but the mesentery is normal except for scattered discrete, moveable, enlarged lymph nodes. Advanced disease is characterized by a contracted, thickened colon without haustration. There may be small telangiectatic vessels (vasa recta) on the serosal surface.

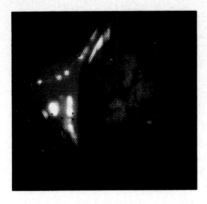

Figure 12–2. Endoscopic appearance of chronic ulcerative colitis.

COMPLICATIONS

Fortunately, most patients only demonstrate symptoms of colorectal involvement of ulcerative colitis. However, the disease may be complicated by a variety of conditions that can affect virtually every area and organ of the body. These will be discussed as local (colonic) and systemic (extracolonic) complications. The list is not intended to be comprehensive. It is quite possible that many extracolonic complications are present in subclinical form and that even the most sophisticated tests fail to reveal them.

Local Complications. According to most authorities, massive hemorrhage requiring hospitalization with transfusions and even emergency colectomy occurs in 3 per cent of patients. Toxic megacolon may occur in 1.6 to 25 per cent of patients. Perforation subsequent to or in the absence of toxic megacolon occurs in 2.8 per cent of patients. Cancer occurs in 1 to 10 per cent of patients, depending on where the statistics were accumulated. The incidence naturally would be higher in hospitals where many resections for advanced cases of inflammatory bowel disease are performed. Benign strictures sometimes cause obstruction of the colon and are found in 9.3 per cent of patients, according to Jackman.

Systemic Complications. Perianal complications such as abscesses, fissures, and fistulas occur in approximately 10 per cent of patients with ulcerative colitis. Arthritis occurs in 20 per cent of cases. Fatty liver and biliary tract disease, bacteremia of the portal system, and cirrhosis are noted in 10 per cent of patients. Phlebitis occurs in 1.2 to 9 per cent, skin lesions in 11 per cent, and ocular lesions in 3.6 per cent of patients. Kidney stones are relatively frequent, occurring in 1 to 6 per cent of people afflicted with this disease. Growth retardation, blood diseases, and a host of other complications may occur. Kirsner provides a complete list of complications.

APPROACH TO THE PATIENT

The patient suffering from ulcerative colitis is usually an intelligent, sensitive young person who may have suffered at one time or other a severe emotional shock. The disease generally is mild to moderate but may be potentially complicated and even life-threatening.

The doctor, therefore, must approach such a patient with sympathy but not pity. Sincere interest and empathy with a positive attitude will go a long way to reassure the patient and ensure his or her cooperation during the thorough and tedious procedures that are necessary to diagnose ulcerative colitis.

DIFFERENTIAL DIAGNOSIS

There are many diseases that exhibit the symptoms of ulcerative colitis. Stool tests, among others, will differentiate the important specific diseases such as amebic dysentery, shigellosis, antibiotic reactions, and gonococcal infection as well as transient or acute gastroenteritis and reactions to enemas and foreign bodies.

ACUTE FULMINATING
ULCERATIVE COLITIS

DIAGNOSIS

History and Physical Examination. In at least 20 per cent of patients, ulcerative colitis has an acute onset. In such cases, the patient is acutely ill and hospitalization is mandatory, since the disease may rapidly progress to the stage of toxic dilatation of the colon. These patients have abdominal cramps, diarrhea, bleeding, fever, and occasionally vomiting. Early in the disease the abdomen is tender and slightly distended. Later there may be more tenderness, guarding, and even signs of peritoneal irritation. A general physical examination is important. Digital examination of the rectum may reveal the finely granular edematous mucosa that is typical of ulcerative colitis. There is usually bloody mucus or feces on the examining finger.

Instrumentation. Proctosigmoidoscopic examination is indicated after a plain film of the abdomen is completed. Examination will reveal the bleeding edematous mucosa, which has the appearance of pink sandpaper. It is not necessary and may be dangerous practice to try to go beyond the rectosigmoid. The danger of perforation is always present when the colon is friable, narrowed, and fixed due to inflammatory bowel disease.

Radiographic Examination. Whenever there is abdominal distention, repeated plain films of the abdomen at three-hour intervals are indicated to rule out toxic dilatation of the colon and even perforation with free air in the abdomen. Dilatation is usually limited to the transverse portion of the colon. Barium enema is contraindicated. Chest x-ray and intravenous pyelogram are indicated.

Laboratory Tests. The white blood count and protein and sedimentation tests are particularly important to monitor this fulminating phase of colitis. Blood cultures, although usually negative, should be taken at the height of the fever.

TREATMENT

Although the following description is for a first attack of ulcerative colitis that has manifested itself as the acute fulminating type, any case of ulcerative colitis may become acutely fulminating. In my experience, the dividing line between the mild to moderately severe and the severe (acutely fulminating) types of ulcerative colitis is the presence or absence of fever. Fever means that the patient is acutely ill and should be treated in a hospital. While I have a wholesome respect for laboratory tests, the history, physical examination, and proctoscopic examination usually can determine which patients need hospitalization.

It is important on admission to the hospital to avoid opiates and atropine-like drugs, which may precipitate or intensify toxic megacolon. Parenteral nourishment, antibiotics, and nasogastric suction, if there is abdominal distention and/or vomiting, are all necessary. Frequent abdominal examination is important to detect the degree of dilatation of the colon. Toxic megacolon is an indication for parenteral steroids. The steroid usually administered is prednisolone in 20 to 40 mg doses given intravenously every 6 hours. Many believe ACTH has absolutely no advantages, although I have seen this drug produce dramatic relief. Surgery is indicated if there is no real improvement in the white cell count, if dilatation of the colon is evident on x-ray in 12 to 24 hours, and especially if the x-ray shows toxic megacolon. Ileostomy with subtotal colectomy is the operation of choice. The rectum is allowed to remain and its proximal end brought out to the abdominal wall as a mucous fistula.

In cases of acute fulminating ulcerative colitis there are four developments which would require emergency surgery: (1) perforation of the colon, (2) toxic megacolon, (3) massive hemorrhage not responding to treatment, and (4) fever, diarrhea, and lowering of blood proteins after four or five days of intensive medical treatment. Ulcerative colitis is notorious for its profound effect on blood coagulability, and patients with massive bleeding seldom leave the hospital without colectomy.

Patients with toxic megacolon who have recovered after medical treatment alone usually have another attack of severe colitis and require colectomy within one year of the initial attack.

CHRONIC ULCERATIVE COLITIS

Chronic ulcerative colitis may be divided into two types, relapsing and continuous. This comparison will facilitate management. Patients with relapsing chronic ulcerative colitis may be symptom-free during intervals between episodes. They are fine for several months, and then, because of a respiratory infection or emotional stress, they experience a flare-up. Patients with continuous chronic ulcerative colitis are never free of symptoms. The physical findings and treatment are different in these two types.

DIAGNOSIS

HISTORY AND PHYSICAL EXAMINATION

The patient usually is aware of the diagnosis of ulcerative colitis and generally has had a work-up elsewhere. Since chronic ulcerative colitis is an unpredictable disease, these patients tend to seek medical attention at various doctors' offices, especially during an exacerbation.

The history usually elicited during an acute phase is that of 5 to 20 loose stools each day containing various amounts of blood. Abdominal cramps and rectal tenesmus or a continuous urge to defecate are symptoms that are always present. Nausea and vomiting are rarely present, but when this is a complaint, the chances are excellent that liver or biliary tract disease is present. One must always remember that chronic ulcerative colitis is primarily a disease of the rectum and colon, and obstruction is a rare complication.

Extracolonic manifestations of this disease must always be considered. Perianal disease is relatively frequent. Lesions occurring on the skin or in the mouth generally indicate low resistance to infection. Clubbing of the fingers and signs of malnutrition usually indicate chronicity. Fever is a sign of severe disease. Tachycardia is likewise a significant sign.

The patient in remission may have few or no symptoms. In fact, constipation rather than diarrhea may be a complaint. However, in these cases there is usually some indication of gross or occult blood. One must always remember that the chief difference between irritable bowel syndrome and colitis is the presence or absence of blood in the stool. The abdominal and proctosigmoidoscopic examinations, which should always be performed, are the only tests which will confirm the diagnosis.

Usually, abdominal examination reveals no significant distention, although deep tenderness along the course of the colon is common. Peristalsis may be prominent, depending on the activity of the disease.

INSTRUMENTATION

In most cases, the result of the proctosigmoidoscopic examination will accurately determine the stage and severity of the disease. It is important to know how much of the rectum or rectum and colon are involved. Most cancer associated with ulcerative colitis occurs in the sigmoid, but it may occur anywhere in the colon. By colonoscopy, it is possible to examine the entire colon and to continue surveillance of the colon for cancer or precancerous changes such as dysplasia. Patients at great risk such as those with long-standing colitis of 8 to 10 years or colitis involving the entire colon should have colonoscopy at 6- to 12-month intervals.

An exciting new concept is evolving from Morson's original work that may allow pathologists to predict which patients suffering from chronic ulcerative colitis are apt to develop cancer. Hyperplastic and other changes in the mucosa known as dysplasia may be found in specimens taken at sigmoidoscopy or colonoscopy. Nugent, Blackstone, and others have performed significant clinical studies to substantiate this concept. In fact, the mucosa overlying a mass lesion of the colon is highly suggestive of the presence of a potential or actual malignancy. Any patient with chronic ulcerative colitis of 8 to 10 years' duration should have yearly colonoscopic examinations with multiple biopsies. Biopsy specimens collected from various parts of the colon should be examined by a pathologist. This constitutes adequate cancer surveillance. Ongoing studies even suggest the possibility of determining which patients are apt to develop cancer merely on the basis of biopsy at the time of proctosigmoidoscopic examination. This may seem unrealistic to us now but the potential is great.

Pseudopolyps, which are common in long-standing disease, are composed of granulation tissue surrounded by ulceration (Fig. 12–3). They are not necessarily premalignant.

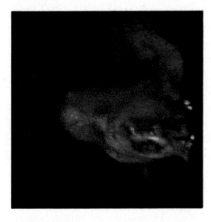

Figure 12–3. Pseudopolyps.

RADIOGRAPHIC EXAMINATION

Barium enema evaluation of the colon will document the extent of chronic ulcerative colitis (Fig. 12–4). It is a good idea to have a colon x-ray as a baseline unless pregnancy or youth makes it undesirable. Some patients may refuse to undergo radiographic examination. Because early mucosal changes may not register positive findings on barium enema evaluation, both x-ray of the colon and colonoscopy are desirable if feasible. The colonoscope and x-ray have proven to be of excellent value both in diagnosis and in evaluating treatment.

TREATMENT

Treatment of chronic ulcerative colitis may vary from no treatment to intense or life-saving measures. It is in direct proportion to the severity and extent of bowel involvement. Eighty-five to 90 per cent of ulcerative colitis patients can be examined and treated on an outpatient basis.

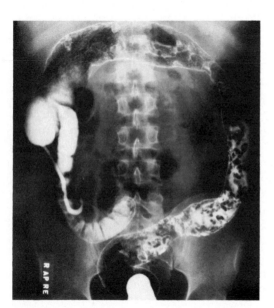

Figure 12–4. Colon x-ray showing pseudopolyposis.

Office treatment consists simply of maintaining proper nutrition, the proper use of sulfa and/or steroid therapy, and recognizing the real indications for surgery.

Nutritional Support

A nutritious and flexible diet is the best "treatment" for chronic ulcerative colitis. Approximately 10 per cent of chronic ulcerative colitis patients have a real or apparent intolerance to lactose. Milk is a good source of protein, and should not be withheld unless intolerance is obvious. When the patient is able to tolerate an adequate diet, the use of supplemental vitamins and weekly injections of vitamin B_{12} is controversial and expensive, and may tend to upset the gastrointestinal tract and therefore interfere with the intake of nourishing foods.

Dietary limitations are only indicated for the acutely ill patient. This and parenteral hyperalimentation has already been alluded to as a preparation for surgery in patients with growth retardation and fistulas. Hyperalimentation similarly has a limited use in ulcerative colitis.

Medical Management

Treatment depends on the extent of involvement of the colon. It is reasonable to treat proctitis with rectal instillations of a foam preparation containing hydrocortisone (Cortifoam) on a daily basis for one week, then gradually decreasing the frequency of treatment by one day each week over a period of six weeks.

Some patients respond to the instillation of sulfasalazine (Azulfidine) suspension in water, using two tablets (1 gm) twice a day for six weeks. This is subject to considerable variation in amounts and frequency, depending on the severity of the proctitis and evidence of response, as determined by weekly proctoscopic examinations. Similar treatment may be given when the rectum and rectosigmoid are involved.

Involvement of the left colon or the entire colon requires Azulfidine by mouth. Usually a dosage of two tablets (1 gm) four times a day is sufficient. Adjusting the proper amount of Azulfidine required for maintenance therapy is similar to regulating the dose of insulin necessary to control diabetes. Every patient must be treated individually. In fact, I am sure that psychologic factors play a great part because some patients do well with one or two tablets daily for one year or more before a flare-up occurs. When a flare-up or exacerbation of the disease occurs, it is best for the patient to resume full therapeutically effective doses immediately. Some patients do well by instituting treatment only for the exacerbations. Others do well on maintenance doses day after day. Treatment should be decided on an individual basis.

Usually an exacerbation requires resumption of sulfa, sedatives, and antidiarrheal drugs by mouth and rectal instillations of hydrocortisone. The latter have the added effect of encouraging the patient to tighten the sphincter to retain the medication, thereby helping to overcome the constant desire for defecation. The patient who does not exercise self-control in this respect will often find that visits to the bathroom may occur every five minutes.

Use of Azulfidine may be potentially dangerous, particularly because of the possible development of side effects such as a low white blood count and allergic reactions. There are many other side effects recorded. Patients may complain of headache or nausea, which is usually relieved by drinking milk with each dose. Sulfa therapy should be monitored by a complete blood count each month during therapy.

Steroids by mouth are indicated only when all other medical treatment has failed. It is best to start with large doses (40 to 60 mg prednisone per day in divided doses); after a few days, when improvement can be expected, the dose can be gradually decreased. As with the Azulfidine, it is well to establish the maintenance dose, that is, the least amount necessary to control the disease.

Steroids should be discontinued as soon as less dangerous drugs such as Azulfidine can be substituted. This may require several weeks to one month, although patients may be kept on steroids for six months or longer if the dose can be kept to 5 or 10 mg prednisone daily. Steinberg suggests that the patient take one mg folic acid daily to prevent macrocytic anemia.

With steroid therapy, all the usual precautions should be taken, such as salt restriction and ample potassium in the form of foods rich in this electrolyte, such as bananas, oranges, and tea. The possible side effects of steroids are numerous, and include electrolyte imbalance, osteoporosis, tetany, fluid retention, diabetes, hirsutism, hypertension, facial edema, "buffalo hump" obesity, psychosis, renal stones, adrenal hypofunction (weakness, hypotension), growth retardation, and lowered resistance to infection. Since 20 to 30 per cent of hydrocortisone enemas are absorbed from the rectum, local side effects may occur after such treatment.

Surgical Management

In dealing with a disease as unpredictable as chronic ulcerative colitis, it is difficult to define indications for surgery that will apply to all circumstances. Table 12–1 lists general situations in which surgery is indicated.

The only cure for chronic ulcerative colitis is proctocolectomy with ileostomy. An increasingly large number of surgeons are establishing a continent ileostomy (Kock pouch). I continue to use the conventional ileostomy (Brooke type), because many are still reporting a 25 per cent incidence of complications associated with the Kock pouch. The Kock pouch is still to be perfected.

A few surgeons preserve the rectum by performing a subtotal colectomy (Fig. 12–5), followed by anastomosis after an interval of 3 to 6 months, during which the rectum is prepared by steroid instillations. If the rectum shows signs of healing, an ileorectostomy is performed. The patients are followed and treated as in the same manner for ulcerative proctitis. However, the inflammatory process in the rectum seldom subsides, and this operation must

Table 12–1. INDICATIONS FOR SURGERY

1. Perforation or impending perforation.
2. Toxic megacolon not responding to medical treatment in three to four days.
3. Massive or recurrent hemorrhage.
4. Cancer or suspected cancer as shown by dysplasia.
5. Stricture with partial or complete obstruction.
6. Extensive anorectal infection.
7. Growth retardation in children.
8. Intractability with inability to work.

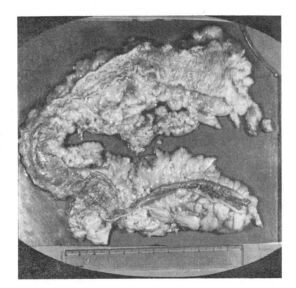

Figure 12-5. Specimen after subtotal colectomy for massive hemorrhage.

stand the test of time. It is a highly selective operation, and many of the patients on whom I performed this procedure needed proctectomy one or two years later because of unacceptable diarrhea or progressive disease. Several patients developed cancer in the retained rectum. However, continued trial or experience with this operation is justified.

More recently at Johns Hopkins, the Mayo Clinic, and other large centers, ileoanal anastomoses are being performed, especially for the very young patient. This must be supplemented by the construction of a pouch in the pelvis and a temporary ileostomy. It is an experimental surgical procedure, but offers hope to the patient who needs colectomy. These operations are contraindicated in patients with Crohn's disease as "pouchitis" and other indications of recurrent Crohn's disease will require removal of the pouch and rectum with construction of the standard ileostomy.

REFERENCES

Bargen, J. A., Chronic Ulcerative Colitis. Charles C Thomas, Springfield, Ill., 1969.

Blackstone, M. O., Riddell, R. H., Rogers, B. H. G., and Levin, B., Dysplasia-associated lesion or mass detected by colonoscopy in long-standing ulcerative colitis: an indication for colectomy. Gastroenterology, 80:366–374, 1981.

Jackman, R. J., Personal communication, 1945.

Kirsner, J. B., Local and systemic complications and associations of inflammatory bowel disease. J.A.M.A., 242:1177–1178, 1979.

Morson, B. C., and Pang, L. C., Rectal biopsy as an aid to cancer control in ulcerative colitis. Gut, 8:423–424, 1967.

Nugent, F. W., Haggitt, R. E., Colcher, H., Kutteruf, G. C., Malignant potential of chronic ulcerative colitis. Gastroenterology, 76:1–5, 1979.

Steinberg, D. M., Allan, R. N., and Thompson, H., et al., Excision surgery with ileostomy for Crohn's colitis with particular reference to factors affecting recurrence. Gut, 15:845–851, 1974.

13

POLYPS OF THE COLON AND RECTUM

INTRODUCTION

Much has been written and said about colorectal polyps. They are common in 6 to 12 per cent of people of all ages. The distribution of polyps in the colon is shown in Figure 13–1. The statistics of Figure 13–1 were determined some years ago, after I had removed about 100 polyps using the colonoscope. All patients had had a colon-x-ray, but not all had had colonoscopy to the cecum. If 5 polyps at the hepatic flexure had been included, there would have been a 10 per cent incidence in the ascending colon. If colonoscopy to the cecum had been performed, as it is in practically all patients today, I believe the incidence would have approached 20 per cent.

Generally speaking, the distribution of polyps in the colon and rectum is similar to that of cancer, in that at least 25 to 30 per cent of polyps and cancer occur in the rectum. Corman has noted a very interesting development: In recent years there have been fewer cases of polyps and cancer in the rectum and more cases in proximal portions of the colon, particularly the cecum. I am certain that this observation could be substantiated in my practice.

Polyps are lesions of all sizes and shapes. Some appear very formidable at first examination, but more detailed observation will frequently show they are attached by a narrow pedicle or pseudopedicle of variable length (Fig. 13–2C and D). The mucosa can be "tented up" when the polyp is grasped by the head for further perusal (Fig. 13–2E), and it is revealed that the pedicle is really attached superficially to the mucosa, which makes removal by electric snare possible. However, there are polyps that are not pedunculated and are attached to the mucosa by a broad base. These are known as sessile polyps and they cause greater concern as to the presence of cancer (Fig. 13–2B). The vast majority of polyps are pedunculated or sessile adenomas and can usually be treated by excision or fulguration. A polypoid cancer may closely resemble a large polyp. Biopsy or multiple biopsies are essential in these cases if the whole lesion cannot be easily removed for the pathologic examination. Even small polyps require biopsy to establish whether they are adenomatous polyps or merely harmless hyperplastic mammilations (Fig. 13–2A). In either case, they should be removed or destroyed by fulguration.

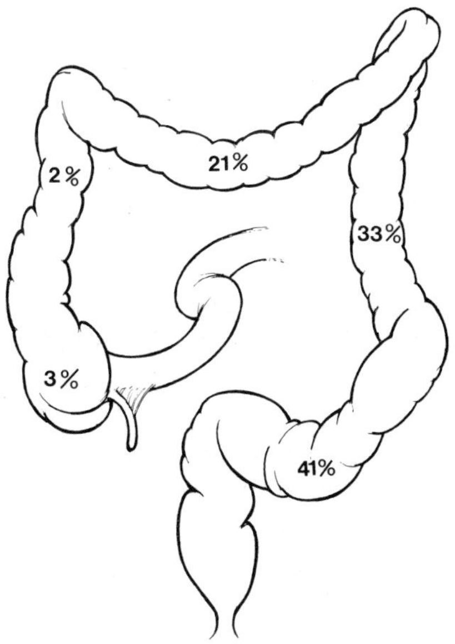

Figure 13–1. Distribution of polyps in the colon (exclusive of rectum).

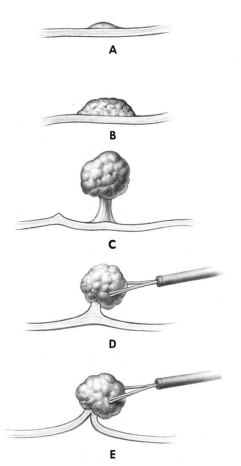

Figure 13–2. Colorectal polyps. *A,* Mamillation. *B,* Sessile. *C,* Pedunculated. *D,* Pseudopedicle. *E,* Tenting.

There are various types of unusual polyps such as congenital, juvenile, and inflammatory. They are different in their behavior and in other characteristics. Even though the unusual polyp is only infrequently encountered, this chapter will include a comprehensive review of them. Thus when they do occur and are recognized and properly treated, a tragedy can be averted.

CLASSIFICATION

The word polyp is a general term used in intestinal disease to indicate any unnatural elevation of tissue that may resemble a tumor. Morson has offered a simple classification of polyps according to both gross and microscopic features. There are four general types: neoplastic, hamartomatous, inflammatory, and unclassified. The neoplastic polyps are further classified according to histology: adenoma (75%), villoglandular adenoma (15%), and villous adenoma (10%).

The adenoma is the most frequently encountered polyp (Figs. 13–3 to 13–6). The consensus among physicians is that they are premalignant. The adenoma may be either pedunculated or sessile and may be pink, red, purple, or the color of the normal mucosa. Although most of these polyps are fairly round and usually resemble small raspberries that may have a stalk or a pedicle, they occur in all sizes and shapes. They vary from a few millimeters to 3 centimeters or larger in size. They may be elongated or have the shape of a keystone or the contour of a strawberry. They may be firm and almost solid. The polyps bleed and may even protrude from the anus occasionally if attached low in the rectum or by a process of intussusception if large and situated in the sigmoid colon. Histologically, the pathologist uses the term tubular adenoma because of the arrangement of the cells in tube-like structures that can be shown by special photography.

The villoglandular polyp (Fig. 13–7) is difficult to differentiate grossly from the adenoma. Because this mixed-type polyp has both adenomatous and villous histologic features, the diagnosis is made by microscopic examination.

The villous adenoma or villous tumor (Figs. 13–8 and 13–9) is indeed a special type of polyp that can be recognized very easily by gross examination, although it may resemble the adenoma. It is essential to realize that this tumor usually is of the same color as normal mucosa and frequently appears in clusters. Many describe this tumor as resembling seaweed because of the many finger-like projections on its surface. It is multicentric in origin and therefore may involve the entire rectum or relatively long segments of the colon.

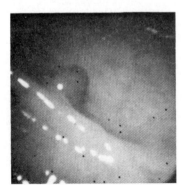

Figure 13–3. Small adenoma.

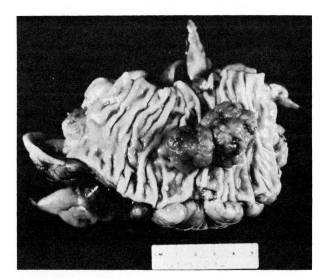

Figure 13–4. Polypoid cancer.

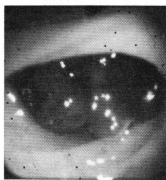

Figure 13–5. Large adenoma.

Figure 13–6. Average-size adenoma.

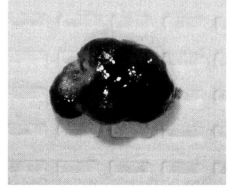

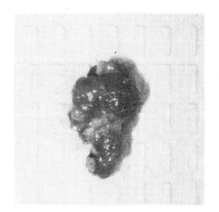

Figure 13–7. Villoglandular polyp.

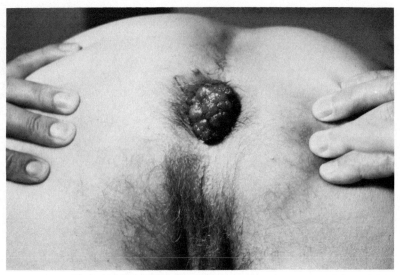

Figure 13–8. Villous polyp prolapsing from anus.

Hamartomatous polyps are non-neoplastic but grossly appear very round and very firm and have an unusually thin pedicle that in juvenile polyps accounts for their frequent spontaneous amputation and extrusion at the time of bowel movement. The pathologist must make the diagnosis. This type of polyp is also seen in the Peutz-Jeghers syndrome. The hamartomas in Peutz-Jeghers syndrome are firm and well anchored in the submucosa and do not usually autoamputate.

Inflammatory polyps (Fig. 13–10), which are also non-neoplastic, are seen frequently in ulcerative colitis where the secondary ulceration has produced islands of inflamed mucosa called pseudopolyposis. Histologically, they are characterized by inflammatory or granular tissue.

The unclassified group of polyps, or hyperplastic polyps, are described by Morson as metaplastic. These are insignificant and rarely are more than 4 mm in diameter. They are sessile and similar in color to the surrounding normal mucosa, and present as tiny bumps on the mucosa. Histologic examination reveals the hyperplasia.

The lymphoid polyps have the gross appearance of slightly enlarged normal submucosal lymph nodes. They appear as myriads of tiny, glistening mucosal cleavations. They must be differentiated from multiple polyposis, which can become malignant. Biopsy quickly makes the diagnosis.

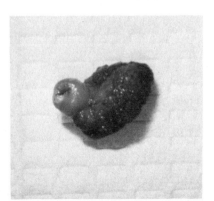

Figure 13–9. Villous polyp.

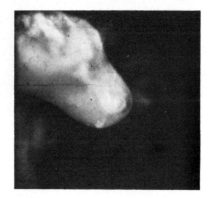

Figure 13–10. Inflammatory polyp.

DIAGNOSIS

When they occur low in the rectum, polyps can be palpated or seen with the anoscope or proctoscope. Polyps situated in more proximal areas can be viewed by x-ray, sigmoidoscopy, or colonoscopy. Chapter 3 contains a detailed discussion of colonoscopy and polypectomy procedures.

DIFFERENTIAL DIAGNOSIS

Differential diagnosis of polyps is relatively simple. A papilla may become enlarged due to irritation or inflammatory reaction of the anorectal area or due to prolapsing internal hemorrhoids. A normal papilla—which is usually 4 mm in diameter—cannot be palpated. When a papilla is even slightly enlarged, the examining finger detects this firm, movable, sensitive structure at the dentate (anorectal) line. If one is enlarged, usually all four or five are enlarged, and they can be palpated as small bead-like structures encircling the anal canal at the dentate line. They may be at a level just within the anal verge or as high as 4 inches above the anal verge in heavy muscular men, depending on the length of the anal canal. Interestingly, when a very large papilla, 1 or 2 inches in diameter, is seen, it is usually single and pedunculated, and therefore usually protrudes from the anal canal upon straining at bowel movement (Fig. 13–11). Just as frequently the papilla prolapses for no obvious reason and must be replaced manually to reduce discomfort.

These enlarged papillae are often clinically mistaken for polyps. If in doubt about the diagnosis, biopsy should be performed, preferably an excisional biopsy if the papilla protrudes. A local anesthetic agent is required for this procedure, since unlike true polyps originating from the mucous membrane, papilla are attached to and covered by skin, and therefore are sensitive.

Polypoid cancers resemble polyps and, except for malignant pedunculated polyps, are sessile. They are firm, but certain adenomatous and all juvenile polyps share this characteristic. A firm indurated or ulcerating area in the stalk of a polyp usually indicates that malignancy in the head of a polyp has extended to the stalk or pedicle.

The differential diagnosis of polyps otherwise consists of the differentiation of the various types of polyps. It is important to recognize the common wart, known as condyloma acuminatum, that occurs in anorectal area as well as the genitalia. External thrombotic hemorrhoids, which occur frequently,

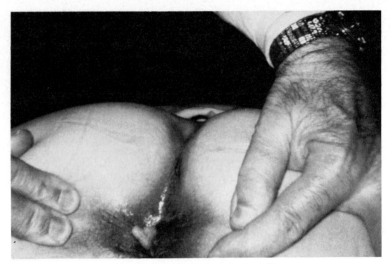

Figure 13–11. Prolapsing papilla.

and internal hemorrhoids, which occur less frequently, should be easily recognized. They usually present suddenly as lumps and are painful when located below the anorectal line.

TREATMENT

Adenomatous Polyps

By all evidence in hand, adenomatous polyps play a vital role in the pathogenesis of rectal cancer. The management of adenomas would be easier if we knew how many years were required for the transition from a benign to a malignant lesion and which polyps would undergo such a change. Prior to the advent of the colonoscope, the practice was that small polyps, e.g., those 1 cm or less in diameter, need not be disturbed and that only large polyps should be removed, since it is thought that polyps less than 1 cm in diameter carry little risk of malignant change. Polyps beyond the reach of the rigid sigmoidoscope posed a treatment dilemma, since they required abdominal surgery for removal. However, with colonoscopy, it is possible to remove or perform biopsy on all polyps regardless of their size and location.

These polyps can and should be removed in the office or outpatient setting utilizing the proctoscope, sigmoidoscope, or colonoscope, depending on the location of the polyp or polyps. For proctosigmoidoscopic examination, the patient has had several enemas, and the rectum and lower sigmoid should be empty. This is important in that if a polyp is seen, it can usually be removed at the initial visit. Removal of polyps involves electrocoagulation or fulguration and requires an empty lower bowel free from flammable gases, such as methane and hydrogen, in order to avoid minor and dangerous explosions. If there is more than a trace of stool, an additional enema can be given in the office before proceeding with fulguration.

Proper fulgurating equipment is so essential in a proctologic office that the important features of such instruments will be discussed in detail. Continuous suction to remove smoke and gases while fulguration is in progress is perhaps the most important principle involved in safe fulguration. One cannot compromise here. A built-in suction device installed by the plumber is ideal. The Buie fulgurating sigmoidoscope is superbly equipped for both examination and treatment. There is a separate opening for the fiberoptic light stick and a built-in suction device to remove smoke. This also makes for efficiency in that it is not necessary to stop fulguration intermittently to remove smoke. A suction "stick" is used at intervals to remove blood, mucus, or water as indicated.

The Hyfrecator with a long electrode or fulgurating stick is satisfactory for fulguration. Many use the special attachment for snaring polyps. The important thing is to understand what you can and cannot do with an electrical unit. Coagulating a piece of beef and coagulating tissue within the intestinal tract are vastly different! However, this is the only way to practice.

You may want to use one instrument for all purposes. However, for convenience and economy, in each treatment room I have Hyfrecators for fulguration and separate units (Neomed and Valley Lab) for snaring polyps. Although coagulation current set at 4 or 5 is used for practically all work, I will occasionally blend the coagulating and cutting currents when shaving polyps in a piecemeal fashion (Fig. 13–12).

The Hirschman anoscope, in various sizes and lengths, is an all-purpose anoscope that may also be used for treating polyps near the anorectal line. When using this anoscope, the overhead light is sufficient except when an area such as a bleeding point in the mid-rectum or higher is to be visualized. In such cases, the light stick provides excellent illumination of the deep recesses of the rectum.

The inverted jack-knife position popularized by Buie is an excellent position for examining and treating the proctologic patient. For this reason, the Ritter table serves admirably for positioning the patient (Fig. 13–13). The actual removal of the polyp is relatively simple (Fig. 13–14). Sessile, flat polyps can be fulgurated at one time or by fractional fulguration, i.e., by burning the polyp at 2-week intervals until it has disappeared entirely. Smaller polyps, those less than 0.4 cm in diameter, can be fulgurated at one

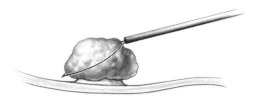

Figure 13–12. Shaving a polyp.

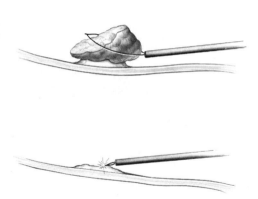

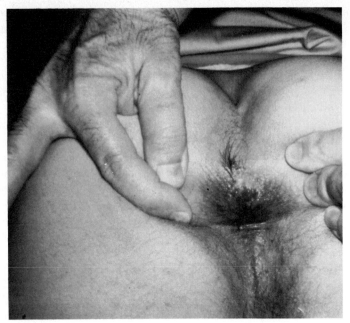

Figure 13–13. Proper placement of patient.

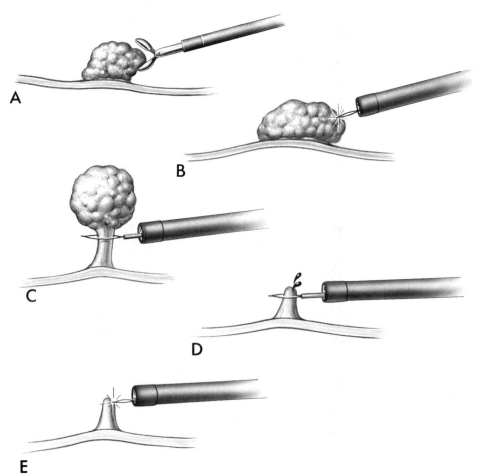

Figure 13–14. Removal of polyp. *A,* Biopsy. *B,* Fulguration. *C,* Snaring. *D,* Bleeding. *E,* Fulgurating bleeding pedicle.

time. If the polyp is pedunculated, the electric snare (Frankfeld) is passed through the sigmoidoscope to an area close to the pedicle of the polyp. The snare is then opened and maneuvered in such a way that the polyp passes through the loop of the snare, which is then partially closed so that the polyp cannot become disengaged. The snare is manipulated so that it is close to the head of the polyp, where the vessels in the pedicle are relatively small. Using only the coagulating current, the snare slowly coagulates or "cooks" across the pedicle. In removing a pedunculated polyp by electrocoagulation of the pedicle, it is important to have the bowel distended. This will prevent the head of the polyp from touching the opposite wall of the bowel, which could cause electrical injury during electrocoagulation. Another way of preventing such injury is to move the polyp quickly back and forth with the snare each time a spurt of current is turned on. It is good practice to cut across pedicles by intermittent spurts of current (Figs. 13–15 to 13–17).

Should bleeding occur after the pedicle is transected, the pedicle can again be snared or lassoed for further electrocoagulation. If this fails, the bleeding pedicle can be treated by coagulation. Bleeding pedicles are no great problem when they are within reach of the sigmoidoscope. When bleeding occurs during colonoscopic polypectomy and the pedicle cannot be snared again, by tedious washings and application of 1:1000 epinephrine to the bleeding area, it is usually possible to stop or slow the bleeding long enough to coagulate the bleeding vessel in the pedicle using the tip of the snare or the hot biopsy forceps.

The size of the artery in the pedicle of these polyps should not be underestimated. They occasionally are 1/5 the size of the pedicle, as observed at open surgery during the precolonoscopic era. In those cases in which a spurting vessel follows colonoscopic polypectomy and in which it is not possible to snare or coagulate the pedicle again, an immediate laparotomy is usually indicated. Pedicles larger than 1 cm in diameter pose a special danger of bleeding immediately following transection; however, there are few true pedicles of this size.

When the polyp is pedunculated, it is relatively easy to secure the entire polyp for pathologic examination. Carcinoma in situ, invasive carcinoma, or

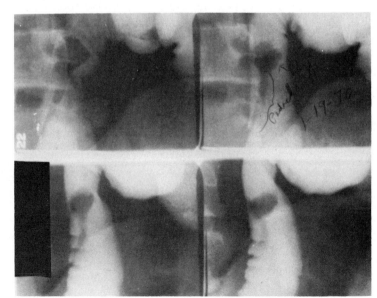

Figure 13–15. Radiograph of a pedunculated polyp.

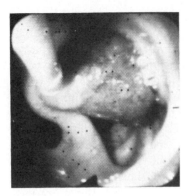

Figure 13–16. Removal of pedicle by electrocoagulation.

extension of the malignancy to the pedicle may be determined, as well as the type of polyp. Many believe that the entire lesion must be removed for pathologic examination. However, such a procedure is not always practical, expedient, or even safe. The advantage of total excision is that not all portions of a polyp are histologically similar. The disadvantages are the possibility of associated bleeding and inaccessibility. For example, a sessile polyp of any size located higher than the rectosigmoid or even the upper portion of the rectum cannot safely be removed by "tenting up" or creating a pedicle by the snare for removal by electrocoagulation.

When the foregoing circumstances prevail, one should rely on the clinical appearance and the results of the pathologic report based on examination of a fragment or fragments of the tissue obtained by fractional biopsy. In fact, several fragments of the polyp can be obtained at one time, leaving only the base of the polyp to be fulgurated. Fractional fulguration, usually at weekly intervals, and intermittent biopsy may also be performed. The frequency of treatment depends on the size of the polyp. I have used this method for many years for the majority of polyps accessible by the proctosigmoidoscope and have no reason to regret this action or abandon the method. A few patients have experienced considerable secondary bleeding approximately a week after a fulguration. Interestingly enough, these patients had bleeding tendencies or were taking aspirin and had surprisingly small sessile polyps no greater than 4 mm in diameter. Perhaps the fulguration was too aggressive, but it is more likely, with the large volume of patients treated, that this complication merely demonstrates the "law of averages," in that not all patients respond identically to any given treatment.

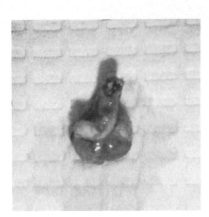

Figure 13–17. Polyp that has been removed.

Villoglandular Polyps. The treatment of this mixed-type polyp is the same as that for the adenomatous polyp.

Villous Polyps

There is no polyp with which the term recurrence has been used more frequently than the villous polyp. I do not believe that a benign polyp will recur after complete removal, but a new polyp may appear. Incomplete excision or fulguration occurs frequently in villous polyps because they are usually of the same color as mucosa and frequently multicentric in the same area. The smaller villous tumors, those less than 2 cm in diameter, should pose no particular problem in treatment, whether they are sessile (as most of them are) or pedunculated.

The chief consideration in treating benign villous polyps is preservation of the rectum. Those of small or moderate size may be fulgurated, regardless of their location in the rectum. When they are situated in the lowermost portion of the rectum, they may be excised by transanal approach. Small ones higher in the colon may be removed by the colonoscope. Some of the moderate-sized ones may be removed piecemeal by this method also.

Larger villous polyps may involve the entire circumference of the rectum. They may be continuous or interrupted by skip areas. If the skip areas are sufficiently wide to permit multiple excisions with closure of the mucosa, there is no problem. If the entire circumference of the upper rectum or bowel is involved, resection with anastomosis is indicated to avoid stricture (Fig. 13–18). Even fulguration of an annular villous polyp results in various degrees of stricture formation when, on those rare occasions, it is performed for a low rectal lesion because a surgical operation will not serve the purpose.

These polyps are attached to the superficial portion of the mucosa, which makes treatment relatively simple. If one took the time to fulgurate these lesions and providing all portions are benign, all of them could be cured. However, in actual practice fulguration of large villous polyps is tedious because of the tremendous amount of mucus present, which makes fulguration difficult.

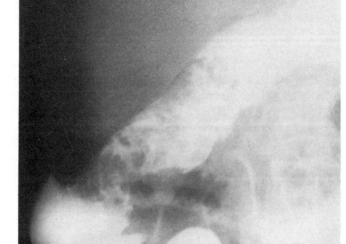

Figure 13–18. "Soapsuds" appearance of large villous polyp.

Large villous polyps in the rectum, especially when they are circumferential, pose the greatest problem. When these are located in the lowermost portion of the rectum, excision by transanal approach is possible. While the risk of rectal stricture is real, this procedure is preferable to sacrifice of the rectum. When large villous polyps are situated high in the rectum, a low anterior resection with anastomosis by hand or using a stapler is the procedure of choice.

Large benign villous polyps in the mid-portion of the rectum pose the greatest problem in treatment. The choice is that of prolonged fulguration or anterior resection with an extremely low anastomosis or pull-through operation. Fortunately, this decision must be made infrequently.

Sometimes the entire rectum is involved with the villous tumor. If it is benign, a pull-through operation should be performed, instead of sacrificing the rectum by the Miles abdominoperineal resection.

LOCAL EXCISION

Mechanical bowel preparation and the inverted jack-knife position are indicated. About the only limitation to local excision of villous tumors of the lower half and even portions of the upper half of the rectum is the size of the anal canal. Local anesthesia is ideally suited for this procedure because of the extent of anal relaxation and hemostasis provided in the area of the tumor. Complete sphincterotomy is seldom necessary, although for tumors situated relatively high in the rectum partial sphincterotomy is indicated. It is futile and potentially dangerous to deliver a polyp with Babcock or Allis forceps from the rectosigmoid area to a lower portion of the rectum. Mucosa tears easily and there is alway the danger of "tenting up" the entire thickness of bowel, especially in a female patient, thereby making it possible to cut full thickness of bowel and enter the abdominal cavity.

Usually tumors selected for surgery in the hospital are sessile and more than 4 or 5 cm in diameter. A Buie hemorrhoidal clamp cannot be placed under the entire polyp for complete excision and placement of interrupted mattress chromic 0 sutures proximal to the clamp. For this reason, a stay suture is placed and the polyp removed with a small margin of normal mucosa one step at a time, i.e., cutting, placing a suture, cutting, etc. Do not underestimate the submucosal plexus, which can bleed briskly and also form hematomas because of inadequate placement of sutures, premature release of clamps, or tearing tissues.

For large tumors near the anorectal line or those which can be brought near the anorectal line by sliding the mucosa, it is well to have a margin of skin for traction. These tumors may involve as much as 75 to 100 per cent of the circumference of the lower rectum. It is especially important to infiltrate the submucosa with a thin layer of local anesthetic agent so that the mucosa can be mobilized easily and as much of the skin of the anorectal line mobilized for traction as is necessary. For support and to avoid secondary complete prolapse, it is usually possible to preserve a portion of the anorectal skin.

After excising the tumor with the excess of mucosa, the proximal edge of the mucosa is approximated to the skin of the anorectal line by interrupted chromic 0 catgut sutures. Postoperative care is similar to that for any minor anorectal surgery (Figs. 13–19 and 13–20).

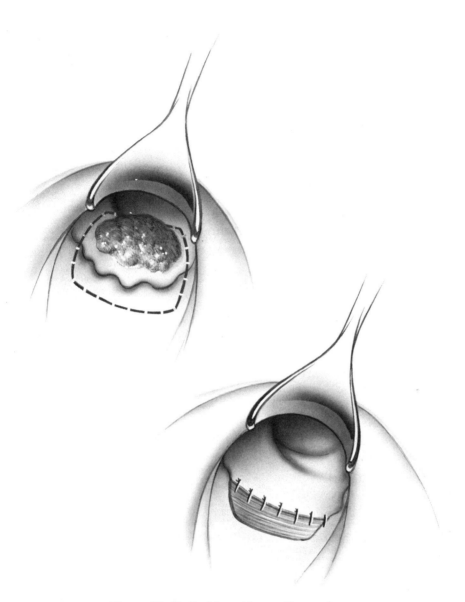

Figure 13–19. Excision of large villous polyp.

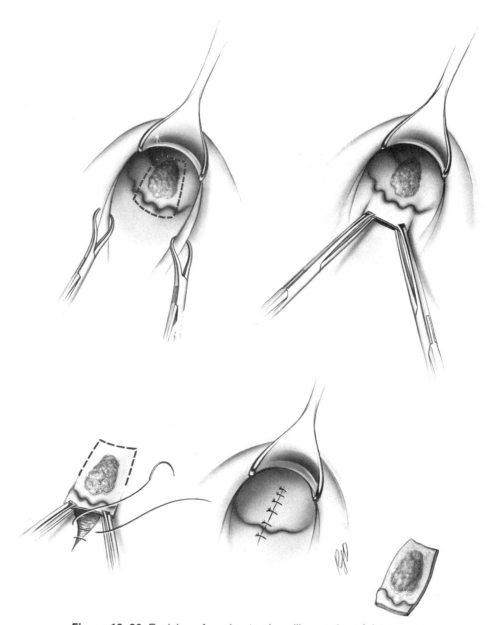

Figure 13–20. Excision of moderate-size villous polyp of the rectum.

Congenital Multiple Polyposis

Congenital multiple polyposis is a general term indicating the presence of numerous polyps in the gastrointestinal tract and certain extracolonic manifestations. As the name implies, the disease is hereditary, and there are various types or syndromes, which will be described under separate headings.

The treatment for congenital multiple polyposis (Fig. 13–21), as in all adenomas, is directed at complete eradication of the polyps to avoid development of cancer. The ideal treatment from this viewpoint would be proctocolectomy with permanent ileostomy, although early reports from a rather limited number of patients indicate that proctocolectomy with ileoanal anastomosis may be the preferred operation when sacrifice of the rectum is necessary. However, there are physiologic consequences of ileoanal anastomosis, or "perineal ileostomy," as some might call it, including diarrhea, incontinence, and skin irritation. This operation has been modified to include a pelvic pouch, which hopefully will resolve these problems.

There are conflicting opinions about the adequacy of rectal-preserving operations. In a study of 143 patients, Moertel et al. found that when the rectal stump is retained, the mortality from cancer in this area increased directly with the length of follow-up. After 25 years, 59 per cent of patients developed cancer, despite frequent proctosigmoidoscopic examinations. However, Harvey et al. of Memorial Sloan-Kettering Cancer Center followed a smaller group of patients who had subtotal colectomy and ileorectal anastomosis. After 26 years, only three patients had developed cancer. These workers believe that rectal preservation is justifiable.

In congenital multiple polyposis, the decision of whether to perform a rectal-saving operation is simplified by the fact that in some patients the rectum is involved with innumerable polyps, to the extent that it is difficult to see areas of normal mucosa. The rectum is literally carpeted with polyps. In Moertel's study, the number of polyps in the rectum at the initial diagnosis influenced the course of the disease, with patients having numerous polyps

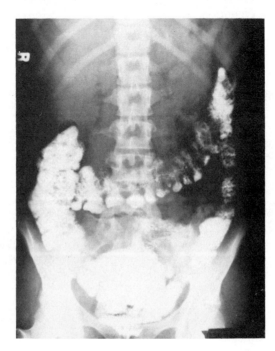

Figure 13–21. Radiographic appearance of multiple polyposis.

exhibiting a tendency toward rectal carcinoma. Such patients will need proctectomy or at least rectal mucosectomy, preferably at the initial operation.

In my opinion, Moertel's observations do not mean that certain patients should not have rectal-preserving operations. There is no doubt in my mind that many patients with congenital multiple polyposis do not and will not need sacrifice of the rectum. In patients with relatively few or easily fulgurable polyps, a rectal-preserving operation should be given a chance, provided that it is feasible to conduct regular sigmoidoscopic examination at 6-month intervals with fulguration of any detected polyps, to insure against development of carcinoma. The studies do emphasize the fact that all adenomas must be destroyed and that lifelong surveillance is the price of rectal preservation.

In male patients, the matter of sexual function must be considered, depending on how much of the rectum is sacrificed. If there are numerous polyps in the rectum, making follow-up by examination and repeated fulgurations difficult, thought should be given to the idea of using ileorectal anastomosis in younger men as a temporary measure until after the period of greatest sexual activity. In an effort to avoid impotence, operations are now being performed in which only the mucosa of the rectum is removed.

Gardner's Syndrome

Sebaceous cysts are removed as they occur or when the patient wants them removed. They are no different from other sebaceous cysts.

Desmoids, which usually occur in the abdominal wall in the area of the incision for the colectomy, are excised widely and generally pose no real problems. The fibromas that may occur in the mesentery of the small bowel may produce obstruction and pose a real problem because of the extent of involvement (Fig. 13–22). It is difficult to remove the fibromas without sacrificing large segments of small bowel, which can result in the numerous problems of short-bowel syndrome and can be life-threatening. In the case illustrated in Figure 13–22, the patient had obstruction of the bowel and excision of the fibromas required removal of most of the ileum. This patient required hyperalimentation in the hospital and at home for a period of years until her body adjusted to the loss of the ileum.

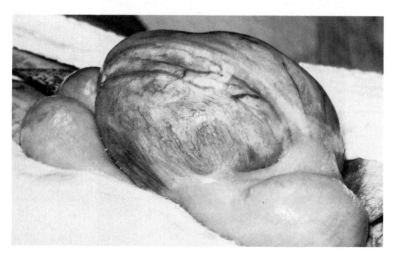

Figure 13–22. Fibroma in mesentery of small bowel.

Peutz-Jeghers Syndrome

Since the polyps in Peutz-Jegher's syndrome are hamartomas, which are benign and have no known malignant potential, operative intervention is limited to those rare cases in which complications such as intussusception in the small bowel occur.

Juvenile Polyps

Because juvenile polyps are hamartomas, which are not premalignant, it is important to differentiate the condition from congenital multiple polyposis. The parents usually bring the child to the office because of rectal bleeding or after noticing a protrusion from the anus. When such a polyp occurs in the rectum, a digital examination can frequently cause the polyp to disengage itself from its very slender pedicle with only slight bleeding. However, it is good practice to coagulate the remaining pedicle if feasible. If the diagnosis is juvenile polyps, any polyps higher in the colon can be ignored, since they will eventually amputate themselves from the stalk and be extruded spontaneously. Some researchers are investigating the significance of these polyps when they occur in certain families and have found hereditary factors that in some respects are analogous to those of congenital multiple polyposis. Since adenomas may be associated with juvenile polyps, it is important to recognize this familial type and remove all polyps in such cases.

Benign Lymphoid Polyps

This is a rather sophisticated name for an insignificant, harmless condition of hyperplastic enlargement of the myriads of lymph nodes found in the submucosa. At first glance, they resemble small polyps. A biopsy will serve to distinguish this condition from polyposis.

REFERENCES

Green, F. L., quoted in Corman, M. L., Colon and Rectal Surgery. J. B. Lippincott, Philadelphia, 1984, p. 249.

Harvey, J. C., Quan, S. H., and Stearns, M. W., Management of familial polyposis with preservation of the rectum. Surgery, 84:476, 1978.

Moertel, C. G., Hill, J. R., and Adson, M. D., Surgical management of multiple polyposis. Arch. Surg., 100:521, 1970.

Morson, B. C., Genesis of colorectal cancer. Clin. Gastroenterol., 5:483, 1976.

14 CHAPTER

DIVERTICULAR DISEASE

INTRODUCTION

The presence of diverticula in the colon was first adequately described in 1849 by Cruveilhier. Subsequently, other researchers noted that the diverticula were occasionally associated with inflammatory changes in the colon, a condition originally called peridiverticulitis but now known as diverticulitis. Extensive studies of autopsy and x-ray material in 1930 showed that 5 per cent of those examined past the age of 40 had diverticula and approximately 17 per cent of these had evidence of inflammation. Incidence gradually increases after age 40, and we now know that for diverticula and diverticulitis the incidence is at least 30 per cent and 25 per cent, respectively. It is doubtful that more than 15 per cent of those with diverticula would show gross evidence of such inflammation.

PATHOLOGY

Diverticula of the colon are outpouchings along the entire colon that represent herniations of the mucosa through the muscle layer of the bowel (Fig. 14–1). The wall of these tiny sacs consists of only serosa and mucosa except at the entrance to these sacs, where a small amount of muscle tissue may be seen microscopically. Diverticula occur where the colon is weakest and that point is between the mesenteric and the lateral taeniae on either side of the bowel, although they may also occur at the antimesenteric border. They are more common in the sigmoid but may occur anywhere in the colon. When diverticula do occur along the entire length of the colon, they are more prevalent in the sigmoid area. They appear as thin, round, soft air bubbles, varying in size from a few millimeters to a half-inch in diameter, that may contain hard stool or fecaliths. It is possible for a person to have from one to hundreds of the acquired type of diverticula in the colon. Since an inverted diverticulum may resemble a polyp, one must always be able to recognize the inverted diverticulum to avoid perforation by erroneous fulguration (Fig. 14–2). However, air insufflation usually causes eversion of the diverticulum, with disappearance of the "polyps."

The congenital type, unlike the diverticula seen in other areas of the gastrointestinal system, is seen rarely in the colon; when it does occur in the

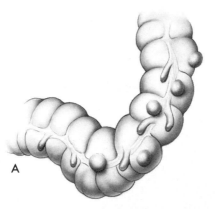

Figure 14–1. *A,* Acquired diverticula. *B,* Congenital diverticulum.

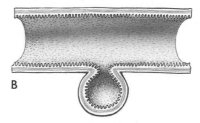

colon, it usually occurs on the right side, although I have seen the so-called giant diverticulum of the sigmoid colon (Fig. 14–3). Some of these large diverticula can be 10 to 20 cm in diameter. The congenital variety naturally contains all of the layers of bowel.

When the diverticula are not inflamed, the condition is called diverticulosis. When the diverticula are inflamed, it is called diverticulitis. It is often difficult to say when diverticulosis ends and when diverticulitis begins. Diverticulitis was originally described as peridiverticulitis or perisigmoiditis. The predominant finding is a thickening of the entire wall of the bowel. Even the fat tags on the bowel or omental tags appear to be enlarged. However, some hypertrophy of the muscle of the bowel is also present in diverticulosis. Whether the inflammation that characterizes diverticulitis is due to gross perforation of the diverticulum or a mere penetration of bacteria through one or more of the diverticula is still to be proven. It would seem logical to assume that a small perforation of a diverticulum would allow inflammation to begin. The finding of one or more intramural abscesses would lend support to this theory. The usual picture encountered is that of a thickened edematous process that may involve most or all of the sigmoid colon, appearing to spread longitudinally in the bowel wall and leaving the mucosa free of disease.

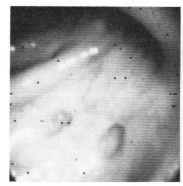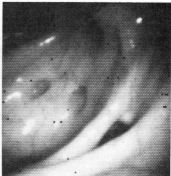

Figure 14–2. Inverted diverticulum.

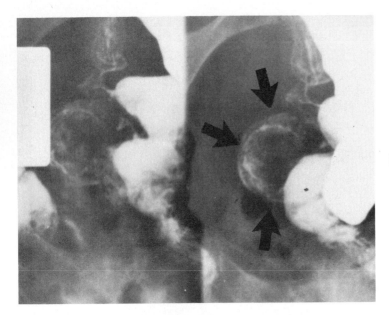

Figure 14–3. Giant diverticulum of the sigmoid colon.

This inflammatory process in the sigmoid can involve any area or any organ in the pelvis and seems to have a natural tendency to agglutinate in other areas. Fortunately, this tendency appears to protect the patient, in that free perforations into the peritoneal cavity are uncommon. Apparently the diverticulum that does perforate is walled off almost immediately by natural processes. It may stick to the wall of the pelvis or to the abdominal wall (Fig. 14–4) or to the bladder or uterus, depending on circumstances. On inspection of the sigmoid in cases of advanced diverticulitis the diverticula are not immediately seen because they seem to be agglutinated in one mass. However, above the area of involvement there are usually other diverticula.

Thus the essential findings in diverticulitis are hypertrophy of the muscular layer and generalized edema of the involved area with a pflegmonous process that appears to fix the sigmoid in the pelvis. There may be an abscess involving most of the pelvis or an abscess between the sigmoid and the uterus, bladder, or vagina. There is a tendency to fistula formation, particularly to the bladder, although fistulas may involve other areas of the large or small bowel, the skin, vagina, uterus, and other organs or tissues. However, these

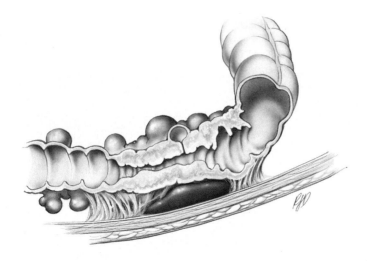

Figure 14–4. Colon attached to the abdominal wall.

fistulas do not occur until rupture of the abscess occurs. Some of these patients will show fistula to the perineum following a rupture of an abscess to this area. Others have reported fistulas to the ureter, although I have not seen this particular condition.

ETIOLOGY

The cause of diverticulosis is not known, although some believe it is due to increased intraluminal pressure with hypertrophy of the muscular coat of the bowel because of hypermotility of irregular spasms along the bowel. These spasms would tend to cause increased pressure in particular areas of the colon, thereby causing diverticula formation. Patients with spastic colon or irritable bowel syndrome with a palpable rope-like sigmoid colon might be considered natural candidates for this disease. However, studies have shown that patients with irritable bowel syndrome are no more subject to diverticulitis than others.

With diverticular disease in Western countries gradually becoming an epidemic, researchers have looked to diet, bowel habits, and general living habits for the answer. Some have attributed the condition to lack of bulk in the diet. There was a time when most colorectal specialists thought that Burkitt was correct in assuming that a high-bulk diet would provide a form of immunity to diverticular disease. However, there are countries in which a traditional high-bulk diet is consumed where there are a considerable number of diverticulitis patients. Thus while high-bulk diets are excellent for general health, they will not necessarily prevent diverticulitis. Constipation, with straining at stool, is also considered a contributing factor; on the other hand, a considerable number of patients with diverticulitis complain of diarrhea.

SYMPTOMS

If diverticulosis alone is present, there are usually no symptoms at all. After a routine barium enema reveals that diverticulosis is present, many patients will develop subjective symptoms such as indefinite or vague abdominal pains that probably have no serious significance. Except for mild cases, which may produce no significant symptoms, diverticulitis presents definite symptoms that vary with the severity of the disease. An acute attack without perforation will produce severe abdominal pain usually in the left lower quadrant because the sigmoid colon is most frequently involved with this disease. Usually there is constipation, although on the other hand there may be slight diarrhea with some distention of the abdomen. Nausea and vomiting usually do not occur. Since diverticulitis causes narrowing of the bowel in the area involved, the pain may be colicky in nature. The patient may notice that he feels feverish. Despite reports in the literature concerning rectal bleeding in diverticulitis, the patients coming under my care have not complained of this symptom.

Patients who develop an intramural abscess from diverticulitis or into the mesentery are apt to have more pain, although such abscesses can occur with very little pain or symptoms other than those of diverticulitis. The usual first attack of diverticulitis or any exacerbation subsides in three to four days. Acute perforation into the peritoneal cavity causes all the signs of generalized peritonitis, which will be discussed later.

DIAGNOSIS

In the presence of diverticulitis without complications, abdominal examination frequently yields pain and guarding, with a palpable thickened, tender sigmoid colon. On sigmoidoscopic or colonoscopic examination, the openings of the diverticula can frequently be seen as slit-like or circular (Fig. 14–5). Frequently, fecaliths will be seen in these openings, although they are best visualized by x-ray examination. It is not always possible to insert the sigmoidoscope for the full 24 cm because of the sacculations and fixation of the lower sigmoid that are typical of extensive diverticulosis. It is sometimes difficult for the radiologist to differentiate cancer from diverticulitis by x-ray examination (Figs. 14–6 and 14–7).

COMPLICATIONS

Perforation. Perforation may occur in diverticulosis and diverticulitis from the administration of an ordinary or a barium enema or following sigmoidoscopic or colonoscopic examination.

Hemorrhage. Hemorrhage caused by diverticulosis is more likely to occur in the elderly patient. Bleeding is apt to occur suddenly, and without warning, the patient will notice blood clots or tarry stool. The patient may lose a unit of blood, and then the bleeding may cease or he may bleed again within months, or even years. The bleeding may also continue intermittently during the first attack until the patient has lost three to five units of blood. The patient may show signs of shock or impending shock. Sigmoidoscopic examination must be performed to rule out a bleeding lesion within reach of this instrument. Generally, however, all that can be seen is a thin coating of dark red to tar-colored blood lining the rectal wall, which indicates that significant bleeding has occurred. If there are clots of blood and evidence of active bleeding, an arteriogram may demonstrate the area of the colon responsible for the bleeding. Vascular deformities in the colon are becoming more frequent in the elderly, and it is surprising how many rare, unexpected lesions can be diagnosed with selective mesenteric arteriography. By skillful placement of a catheter in a femoral artery and advancement to the superior and inferior mesenteric arteries, the dye can be injected to study the branches of these vessels by means of x-ray. Naturally, such examinations should precede the barium enema.

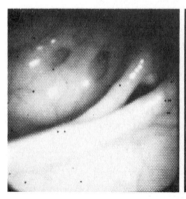 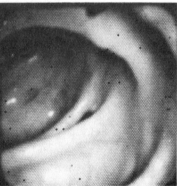

Figure 14–5. Diverticulum as seen through a colonoscope.

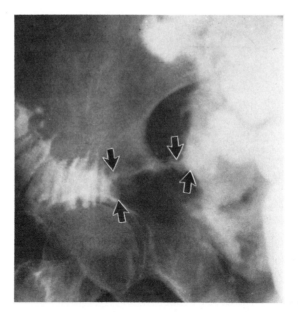

Figure 14–6. X-ray demonstrating similarity between diverticulum and cancer.

Intestinal Obstruction. In spite of the fact that diverticulitis of the sigmoid colon produces narrowing, intestinal obstruction is not a frequent problem (Fig. 14–8). It is very important to rule out small bowel obstruction, because diverticulitis can extend by an inflammatory process to portions of the small bowel and cause mechanical obstruction (Fig. 14–9).

Fistula Formation. Between 4 and 23 per cent of diverticulitis patients show a colovesical fistula (Fig. 14–10). This wide range of incidence may be explained by the fact that some institutions see more of this disease than others. The patient usually makes the diagnosis or provides the symptoms that lead to the diagnosis because of bladder symptoms. Occasionally, the

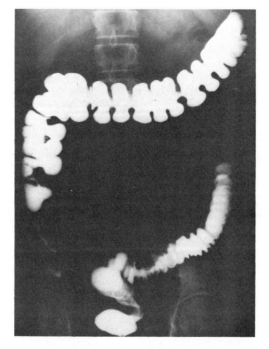

Figure 14–7. X-ray showing narrowing of colon.

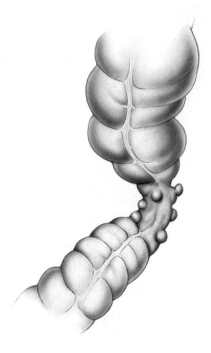

Figure 14–8. Area of diverticulitis causing obstruction.

patient will complain of passing air through the urethra. This type of fistula can also be caused by cancer of the colon or rectum, or by Crohn's disease.

Sigmoidoscopy occasionally and colon x-ray frequently demonstrate the fistula. Cystoscopy is usually ordered, but seldom can the actual fistula be visualized, and the urologist's findings may be limited to the appearance of cystitis or a tuft of granulation tissue in an area in the bladder highly suspicious of inflammatory process or fistula. Although indicated, an intravenous pyelogram seldom reveals the fistula.

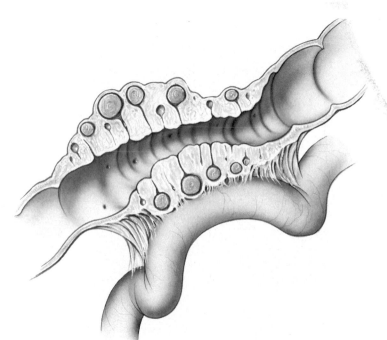

Figure 14–9. Inflamed colon attached to a segment of the small bowel.

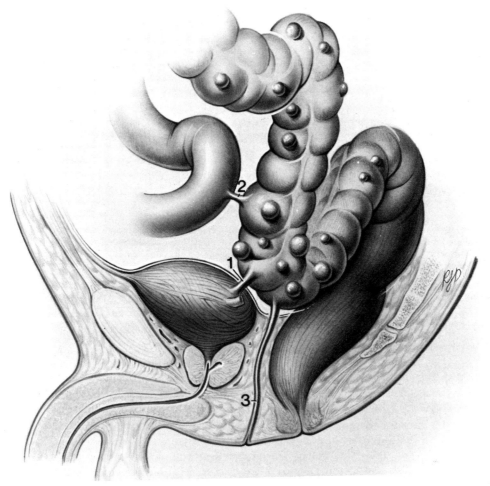

Figure 14–10. Fistulas to the bladder *(1)*, small bowel *(2)*, and perineum *(3)*.

TREATMENT

As indicated in Table 14–1, the management of diverticulitis depends on the course of the disease. Asymptomatic diverticulosis does not require treatment. The abdominal symptoms are usually vague in these cases, and the patient needs a great deal of reassurance. While a high-residue diet is indicated, it should be nonirritating; for example, strawberries, raspberries, and blackberries are prohibited because of their sharp seeds. The use of laxatives and the habit of straining at stool are to be avoided. If the patient cannot eat enough bulk in the diet, supplemental bulk can be provided by psyllium hydrophilic mucilloid preparations such as Metamucil, Konsyl, and similar products.

The first attack of acute diverticulitis without complications should be treated medically, although many report recurrence rates up to 50 per cent within two years after the first attack. The treatment of the first attack of diverticulitis consists of bed rest, a clear-liquid diet, administration of a drug such as meperidine (Demerol) for pain, short courses of antibiotics, intravenous fluids, and occasionally a Levin tube if nausea appears to be a problem. Careful observation is necessary, because the first attacks of acute diverticulitis occasionally lead to perforation of the bowel and abscess formation.

Table 14–1. MANAGEMENT OF DIVERTICULAR DISEASE

Diagnosis	Treatment
Diverticulosis	High-fiber diet
Acute diverticulitis (first attack)	Medical
Recurrent diverticulitis	Segmental resection
Intramural and/or mesenteric abscess	Segmental resection
Pelvic abscess	Hartmann resection
Abscess and diffuse pelvic inflammation	Drainage and colostomy
Free perforation into peritoneal cavity	Hartmann resection
With small bowel involvement	Segmental resection of colon and small bowel
Massive hemorrhage (first attack) not requiring over 4 units of blood	Medical
Persistent hemorrhage	
From identified area of colon	Segmental resection
From unidentified area of colon	Subtotal colectomy with ileorectal anastomosis
Obstruction (partial)	
When bowel can be prepared	Segmental resection
Obstruction (complete)	Hartmann resection or colostomy only
Colovesical fistula	Segmental resection and closure of fistula
Colovaginal fistula	Segmental resection

After a few days of suitable treatment, the temperature and white blood count return to normal, and if bowel function is satisfactory, the diet can be increased to first a soft diet and then a regular diet over the course of several weeks.

During the acute attack it is important to avoid manipulation of the bowel by sigmoidoscope and barium enema. These procedures have been known to cause complications. A few weeks after the subsidence of symptoms, sigmoidoscopic examination and barium enema may be performed with caution in order to make a definite diagnosis. In diverticulitis of the sigmoid colon of any degree, it is usually impossible to insert the sigmoidoscope much above the rectosigmoid. These procedures give the physician the opportunity to estimate the amount of normal bowel below the disease, which is important if resection becomes necessary.

Diverticulitis usually recurs within the first two years. Recurrent attacks accompanied by radiographic changes in the colon, such as narrowing and thickening of the bowel wall, especially if there are many diverticula in the sigmoid, suggest the need for resection of the involved portion of the colon. Thus when the patient has had recurrent attacks and the diagnosis is well established, the treatment is surgical. Following suitable preparation of the patient, sigmoidectomy in one stage is the usual procedure. Because of the inflammatory nature of the disease, anastomosis of the bowel may be complicated. At laparotomy, there is usually a fusiform-shaped inflammatory mass lying in the cul-de-sac, which may be adherent to the various areas in the pelvis and which at first may seem impossible to resect. However, when freeing the adhesions carefully from the various structures of the pelvis, such as the bladder or uterus, and the lateral walls of the pelvis, it is surprising how often the mass comes up easily to the abdominal wall. It is important to free the bowel and even the rectosigmoid so that soft, pliable, normal rectosigmoidal bowel is available inferiorly and superiorly. I seldom free the splenic flexure for sigmoidal diverticular disease, although I do free the lateral peritoneal reflection up to the spleen to give some mobility to the descending colon. There must be ample bowel on either side, so that when the anastomosis is completed the entire anastomotic area falls into the pelvis without tension. Interrupted five 0 wire interrupted sutures are used. Wire is superbly suited for inflammatory conditions of the bowel, since it produces practically no reaction around the area of anastomosis. It is important to remove all of the diverticula below the resection, but it is not necessary to remove all the diverticula above the area of resection. It is important not to place sutures through a diverticulum. Both ends of bowel to be anastomosed must be completely free of disease. It is not necessary to close the floor of the pelvis. Two Penrose drains are placed in the pelvis and brought out through a separate stab wound, and these are normally gradually shortened over a period of three to seven days following surgery. A lower midline incision, which can be extended above the umbilicus as necessary, has proved very satisfactory. As in all abdominal surgery, incidental appendectomy is performed if convenient.

ABSCESS FORMATION AND FREE PERFORATION

If after four or five days there is no significant improvement and especially if there is evidence of a mass in the left lower quadrant that is enlarging and there are indications of abscess formation, the decision of whether to perform immediate surgery must be made. There are some surgeons who would wait for the abscess to "point," either to the skin, the rectum, or the vagina. However, if digital examination of the rectum does not show any signs of induration and fluctuation, and vaginal examination does not show such findings except for the usual induration that occurs in diverticulitis of the sigmoid, it might be a safe procedure to procede with immediate laparotomy rather than to wait for signs of generalized peritonitis. If at laparotomy there is no sign of an abscess formation, one can procede with a routine sigmoidectomy for diverticulitis, as already described (Fig. 14–11). If an intramural abscess is found in the colon or between the leaves of the mesentery in the area of the diverticulitis (Fig. 14–12), it may be possible to excise the involved bowel and mesentery without opening the abscess. On the other hand, if the abscess is attached to the pelvic wall or cul-de-sac, it may be necessary to drain the abscess, flush the pelvis with povidone-iodine (Betadine) or a similar solution, and procede with the removal of the diseased segment of sigmoid.

In the presence of a pelvic abscess, one must be cautious about performing a primary anastomosis, and a Hartmann procedure should be used. The Hartmann procedure is a two-stage operation that in the first stage removes

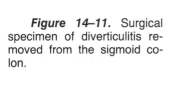
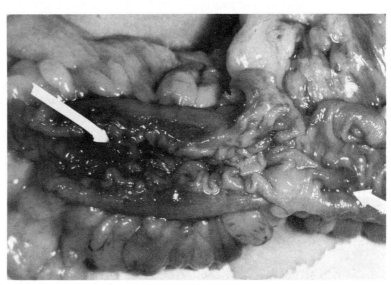

Figure 14–11. Surgical specimen of diverticulitis removed from the sigmoid colon.

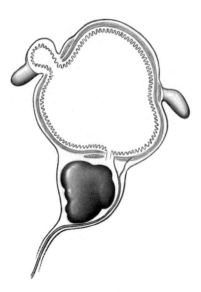

Figure 14–12. Abscess between leaves of mesentery.

the sigmoid involved with diverticulitis and leaves a normal rectal stump that can be later used for an anastomosis. Colostomy is performed through a separate wound and the rectal stump closed with 00 chromic sutures, although wire sutures may also be used. Blow-out of the rectal stump has been reported frequently in the literature, but this probably does not occur unless one attempts to close an edematous rectal wall. The sump type of drain is used in the pelvis along with Penrose drains. The sump drain can usually be removed in a few days, but the Penrose drains should remain for as long as there is any drainage other than serous.

The second stage of the Hartmann procedure consists of taking down the colostomy and performing an anastomosis of colon to rectal stump. Nunes and colleagues perform the second and final stage two to three months after the initial resection. They report a mortality rate of 8 per cent utilizing the Hartmann procedure for complications of diverticulitis.

There are some who believe the Hartmann procedure can be used in practically all patients with pelvic abscesses or free perforations due to diverticular disease. It has been my experience that in some patients with diffuse inflammation in the pelvis with abscess from diverticular disease, it is necessary to occasionally back away from primary resection. I do not hesitate to drain the pelvis freely and perform a transverse colostomy rather than to proceed with a difficult and tedious dissection of the rectosigmoid with the dangers of injury to the ureter, bleeding, and other iatrogenic effects. Although primary resection is preferred and many report mortality up to 40 per cent for the staged procedure without primary resection, Classen and associates from Johns Hopkins Hospital report an overall mortality rate of 11 per cent for the staged procedures (three-stage procedure).

Wound infection is the most common complication following resections for perforating diverticulitis. In my practice, the abdominal wound is closed with single-layer interrupted through and through wire sutures. The peritoneum and fascia are included with each suture. The wound is flushed with Betadine, and the skin is closed with interrupted wire or Prolene sutures. Telfa wicks saturated with Betadine are inserted between the skin sutures every inch or two along the incision. The wicks are left in the subcutaneous tissue for a least three or four days. This method of abdominal wall closure and drainage is used in all cases of colorectal resections. In all operations for complicated diverticulitis where there is abscess formation or free perforation with peritonitis, antibiotics must be chosen to cover both aerobic and anaerobic organisms.

Free perforations into the peritoneal cavity are frequently but not always diagnosed by the flat plate of the abdomen showing free air under the diaphragm. For sigmoid diverticulitis with perforation, the Hartmann procedure has become the first choice of treatment. Free perforation associated with shock, which indicates gram-negative infection, is a bad prognostic sign, and usually means there is gross fecal contamination of the peritoneal cavity.

MASSIVE HEMORRHAGE

Massive hemorrhage occurs chiefly in the elderly. Subtotal colectomy with ileorectal anastomosis procedure is curative and is well tolerated even in elderly patients. Mesenteric angiograms can often localize the source of bleeding, thus enabling the surgeon to perform a more limited resection of the bowel. If the bleeding point is found in either side of the colon—and massive bleeding usually occurs from diverticula in the right colon—the appropriate hemicolectomy should be performed. I personally am very cautious about performing left or right hemicolectomy for massive hemorrhage when the exact location of the bleeding point has not been definitely demonstrated.

It is not always necessary to perform surgery for the first episode of massive hemorrhage from diverticular disease, since it frequently subsides with several blood transfusions and other appropriate care. Bleeding may never recur, although if it does recur, it is within the 12-month period following the initial episode. Emergency subtotal colectomy for bleeding is indicated when the bleeding persists after four or five units of blood have been given. Usually the decision for operation is made within 12 hours of admission.

OBSTRUCTION

The most common complaint of patients presenting with complicated diverticular disease of the sigmoid are symptoms relative to obstruction. If after thorough examination obstruction is the sole complaint and the only finding, the bowel can be suitably prepared for an elective operation. If preparation is not satisfactory and the obstruction not relieved, the decision of what to do must be made at the time of laparotomy. The sigmoid must be carefully explored as well as the surrounding small bowel. If the colon is tremendously dilated, it might be well to consider resection without primary anastomosis. An anastomosis can be extremely dangerous in the presence of high-grade bowel obstruction. In these rare cases, a preliminary colostomy is indicated if primary resection cannot be done at the same time.

FISTULA FORMATION

Fistulas do not usually cause a great problem for the surgeon. A colovesical fistula, depending on what stage it is seen, may merely be a fibrous-like tube with small area of induration around the bladder. After removal of the sigmoid and detachment of the bladder, especially if the opening is well up on the dome where there is ample bladder for resection, it is good practice to remove the hard fibrous tissue of the bladder wall so that one has soft pliable bladder to close using 00 chromic catgut interrupted sutures. If the fistula

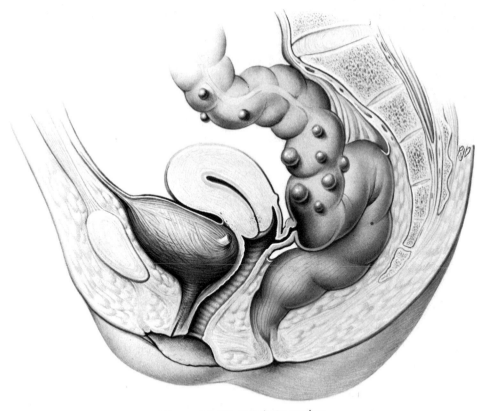

Figure 14–13. Fistula to vagina.

involves the small bowel, it is usually necessary to resect the segment of bowel and perform a primary end-to-end anastomosis. Colocutaneous and colovaginal fistulas (Fig. 14–13) heal spontaneously after the affected sigmoid is removed. It should be emphasized that it is not necessary to do a three-stage procedure simply because of the presence of a fistula.

OTHER AREAS OF THE COLON

The diagnosis of diverticulitis of the right colon is especially difficult. The condition usually presents as an acute abdomen or appendicitis. A simple diverticulum on the right side of the colon may perforate following a barium enema. Prior to surgery, a perforating carcinoma cannot always be ruled out. According to most reports in the literature, a right colectomy is necessary for extensive diverticulitis of the right colon.

REFERENCES

Burkitt, D.P., Walker, A.R.P., and Painter, N.S., Effect of dietary fiber on stools and the transit-times, and its role in the causation of disease. Lancet, 2:1408, 1972.

Classen, J.N., Bonardi, R., O'Mara, C.S., et al., Surgical treatment of acute diverticulitis by staged procedures. Ann. Surg., 184:582, 1976.

Cruveilhier, J., Traité d'Anatomie Pathologique, Vol. 1. Paris, Boillière, 1849, p. 593.

Goligher, J.G., Surgery of the Anus, Rectum and Colon, 4th ed. London, Baillière Tindall, 1980, p. 881.

Nunes, G.C., Robnett, A.H., Kremer, R.M., and Ahlquist, R.E., Jr., The Hartmann procedure for complications of diverticulitis. Arch. Surg., 114:425, 1979.

Rankin, F.W., and Brown, P.W., Diverticulitis of the colon. Surg., Gynecol., and Obstet., 50:836, 1930.

CHAPTER 15

CANCER

INTRODUCTION

Colorectal cancer is the most common internal cancer of the Western world. The disease is of unknown etiology and its behavior is only partially predictable. The purpose of this chapter is to summarize the limited information concerning this complex disease by reviewing the literature and my own experience in dealing with 1600 consecutive patients suffering from this disease. The office procedures helpful in prevention and early diagnosis of the common types of malignant and premalignant lesions will be described, as well as the principles and technics of treatment. This text is not meant to be a detailed exposition of the classification, research, and management of colorectal cancer; it is a review of essential information.

PATHOLOGY

Some years ago, I reviewed 684 consecutive colorectal cancers in an effort to determine the frequency and types of tumors involved (Table 15–1). The vast majority of cancers were found to be *adenocarcinomas*. These tumors are of various sizes and show various degrees of penetration of the bowel wall and various degrees of involvement of the circumference. Most adenocarcinomas are of the ulcerated type (72 per cent); the remainder are polypoid (20 per cent), mucoid (5 per cent), and scirrhous (3 per cent).

Table 15–1. CANCER OF THE COLON, RECTUM, AND ANAL CANAL

Type	Number	Per Cent
Adenocarcinoma	667	97.51
Squamous cell carcinoma	8	1.17
Cloacogenic (basaloid) carcinoma	3	0.44
Lymphosarcoma	2	0.29
Melanoma	2	0.29
Basal cell carcinoma	1	0.15
Leiomyosarcoma	1	0.15
	684	100

There is nothing that "feels" quite like a cancer. It is rock-like, but unlike a piece of hard stool it is attached to the wall of the colorectal area. It can be moved slightly or moderately, depending on the degree of penetration of the bowel wall. If the tumor is attached to the prostate, sacrum, or other fixed structure, it is not movable and the term fixed is frequently used to describe it.

Ulcerated adenocarcinomas grow and raise themselves above the mucosa and eventually outgrow their blood supply, thereby causing ulceration or necrosis. The blood supply tends to be better around the periphery of the tumor, and therefore the edges of the tumor tend to be higher and prominent and the center or the tumor depressed or umbilicated. The tumor can be recognized by palpation, if within reach of the finger, by visualization at endoscopy, and by barium enema examination. Various degrees of involvement of the circumference of the bowel can be ascertained by the finger. A good rule to follow is to recognize that approximately 18 months are required for a tumor to encircle the rectum or bowel.

Polypoid adenocarcinomas are not ulcerated but raised tumors that vary in size but are always firm to the touch. They are not generally as firm as the ulcerated type and tend to grow towards the lumen of the bowel, therefore appearing higher than the ulcerating type.

Mucoid adenocarcinomas, although ulcerating, are characterized by more mucus secretion than the other types, and are also known as mucinous or colloid adenocarcinomas. They are sometimes referred to as signet-ring cell cancer, because on histologic examination the columnar cells are filled with mucus to such an extent that the nucleus is literally pressed to the base of the cell, creating the appearance of a signet ring.

Scirrhous ulcerating adenocarcinomas constitute approximately 3 per cent of the adenocarcinomas and are characterized by relatively long involvement of the bowel; the average length of these tumors is 8 cm. They are also characterized by fibrous contraction, as in linitis plastica of the stomach. These tumors are more apt to occur in older individuals and tend to obstruct the bowel.

Polypoid carcinomas have the best prognosis; mucoid type tends to be highly anaplastic and has the worst prognosis. Ulcerating and scirrhous adenocarcinomas have a prognosis somewhere between the other two types.

Relatively Infrequent Cancers

Some years ago I reviewed 25 consecutive primary cancers of the anal canal, including one each of the following rare tumors—Bowen's disease, leiomyosarcoma, adenocarcinoma arising in an anal duct, and basal cell tumor—and two melanomas. The remaining tumors were squamous cell cancers or variants.

The *carcinoid* is a low-grade malignancy that may even be benign in many cases. Carcinoid tumors are so rare that it is difficult to prove statistically any general statements made about them. They were described in 1928 by Masson, who believed that the tumors arose from the Kulchitsky cells at the base of the glands of Lieberkühn. The cells, which are thought to be of entodermal origin, have an affinity for silver stains; hence the growths are also termed argentaffinomas. The Kulchitsky cells also secrete serotonin. Under certain circumstances such as massive metastases to the liver, large amounts of serotonin are secreted by the tumor and serotonin derivatives may be found in the urine. High levels of serotonin may be responsible for the carcinoid syndrome—skin flushing, diarrhea, constriction of the bronchi, and a rise in pulmonary pressure.

Carcinoids are occasionally found as an incidental finding at laparotomy. They present in the early stages as a white or yellowish nodule or nodules in the appendix or in the small bowel, where they may be multiple. The next most frequent site is the rectum. They are seldom over 2 cm in diameter and may ulcerate, making it difficult to differentiate them grossly from adenocarcinomas.

Lymphosarcoma is an exceedingly rare tumor. While tumors of this type are seen as a part of generalized disease, I have seen only three considered as primary tumors. In 1500 cases of colorectal cancer Goligher has seen only two patients suffering from this disease, both with lymphosarcoma of the rectum. According to Jackman and Beahrs the most common site is the ileocecal area, although the tumor may occur anywhere in the gastrointestinal tract. When found in the colon or rectum, there is a 50 per cent chance that it is secondary to generalized lymphosarcoma.

According to Stearns there are four types of lymphosarcoma: lymphosarcoma, reticulum sarcoma, giant follicular lymphosarcoma, and Hodgkin's disease. The reticulum sarcoma is the most common. The lymphosarcomas I have seen involved the submucosal tissues of the entire bowel wall, which was thickened with enlarged lymph glands in the mesentery of the involved bowel. The lesions resembled Crohn's disease without the rake-like ulcers. The mucosa was thickened and edematous. On seeing the gross lesion, the impression is that of generalized involvement of all layers of the bowel and the lymph nodes, in contradistinction to an adenocarcinoma or a leiomyosarcoma. Biopsy may be necessary to confirm the diagnosis.

Leiomyosarcoma is a malignant smooth-muscle tumor that remains localized or apparently remains localized until it ulcerates through the mucosa. These tumors spread primarily by the blood stream. Leiomyosarcomas are frequently mistaken for benign leiomyomas. Submucosal leiomyomas are relatively common, benign smooth-muscle tumors of the gastrointestinal tract. As expected, they feel like muscle and are well localized. Their most common site is the stomach. It is difficult to state if and at what point in time or size leiomyomas become malignant. I have seen a large leiomyoma of the rectum, 6 cm in diameter, that appeared perfectly benign. Local excision was performed, the pathologist found no evidence of malignancy, and the patient did well.

Leiomyosarcomas are frequently large lesions. Figure 15–1 illustrates a massive tumor involving the entire left buttock. Small tumors, those less than 2.5 cm in diameter, do well with local excision, especially if performed before ulceration through the mucosa occurs. The larger ones do poorly regardless of how radical the attempt at cure.

Basal cell carcinoma, or rodent ulcer, rarely occurs at the anal area. Only five such patients were seen at Memorial Hospital in the past 25 years. The tumor has distinct rolled edges with a central shallow ulceration, as seen in similar but more frequent tumors of the face. It does not invade deep structures and will not metastasize. The pathologist has no difficulty making the diagnosis. Local excision is sufficient.

Another rare tumor, *perianal Paget's disease,* presents as a pale grey, crusty, plaque-like lesion that may or may not be inflamed. Pathologic diagnosis shows Paget's cells—large, single, intraepithelial cells, whose pale cytoplasm stains positively with aldehyde-fuchsin stain—as a prominent

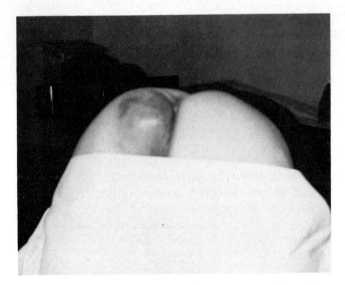

Figure 15–1. Large leiomyosarcoma of the buttock.

feature. In this manner, the disease is distinguished from Bowen's disease. An underlying adenocarcinoma may be present, and the extent of its invasion or involvement of lymph glands determines the prognosis.

Bowen's disease may manifest itself as a reddish, scaly, plaque-like area at the anal verge. The differential diagnosis includes extramammary Paget's disease, keratosis, and basal cell carcinoma. The underlying pathology is that of an intraepidermal squamous cell cancer. The Bowen cell is pathognomonic for this condition.

Unfortunately, as Figure 15–2 shows, these lesions can be extensive when first seen. A high index of suspicion is necessary if one is to make an early diagnosis of these extremely rare lesions. The important sign is localized induration. Many patients will present for treatment for the various eczema-like manifestations of idiopathic pruritis ani. In these cases, there is generalized thickening and frequent lichenification of the skin. One must be alert to anything unusual, for example, a localized area that is somehow different from the surrounding area. An early biopsy of the affected area may save a life, since invasive squamous cell carcinoma can quickly occur.

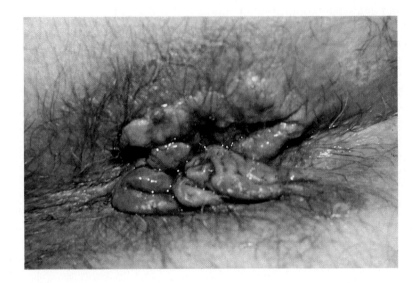

Figure 15–2. Advanced Bowen's disease of the anal canal.

In a series of 4000 anorectal cancers at St. Mark's Hospital, Morson states that only 10 were *melanomas*. These tumors arise from the melanoblasts of the skin, although many tumors at the anal verge or in the anal canal are unpigmented. Any nodule, atypical-looking external hemorrhoid, or ulcer with a deep-red to black color should arouse suspicion as to the presence of melanoma.

Frequently, these "ulcers" are merely breaks or abrasions in the skin overlying an external hemorrhoid with slight secondary infection. My experience has shown that an abrasion usually looks exactly as if one had deliberately torn the thin skin over the hemorrhoid. There is no thickening or semblance of nodularity. Furthermore, a subcutaneous hematoma is painful if seen during the first few days, is movable, and will show the appearance of discoloration through the skin typical of an external thrombotic hemorrhoid.

The history is extremely important, especially if the lesion resembles an external thrombotic hemorrhoid. Of diagnostic importance is that melanoma is neither painful nor instantaneous in its occurrence. Inspection with excellent illumination and palpation are the key words to lead the way to early diagnosis of these rare tumors. Anything that looks like or feels like an ulcer or nodule should be inspected very closely. If there is reasonable doubt, a biopsy, preferably a complete excisional biopsy under local anesthesia, should be performed. I have been able to diagnose early squamous cell carcinomas in this manner.

Squamous cell cancer of the colon, although rare, can occur by a process of metaplasia. Ulcerative colitis and adenomatous polyps are the two main sources of this change. This disease should not be confused with squamous cell tumor of the anal canal. In referring to cancers of the anal canal Goldberg indicated quite aptly that since there is no uniform terminology, it is difficult to interpret the results of treatment. He is apparently referring to squamous cell carcinoma (Fig. 15–3) and its variants basaloid carcinoma, mucoepidermoid carcinoma, transitional-cell carcinoma, and cloacogenic carcinoma, as well as basal cell carcinoma, which is a separate and distinct entity.

Tumors of the perianal area, anal verge, and anal canal require expert surveillance, both macroscopically and microscopically, and good judgment on the part of the clinician to decide on proper diagnosis and treatment (Fig. 15–4). Generally speaking, the pathologist must make a diagnosis of cancer,

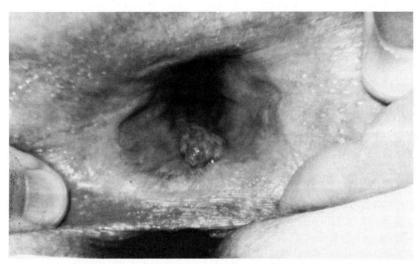

Figure 15–3. Squamous cell cancer of the anal canal.

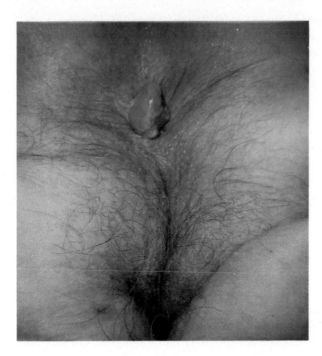

Figure 15–4. Adenocar-cinoma arising in an anal duct.

in which case it will be the squamous cell cancer or one of its variants. The only exception to this would be in patients having an adenocarcinoma in the lower rectum which is invading the anal canal (Fig. 15–5).

Careful inspection of the gross characteristics of the tumor is not only important for diagnosis but for determining the nature of the treatment indicated. The size of the tumor, its location and the depth of penetration, and particularly the distance between it and the dentate line are important. These characteristics are particularly important in selecting local excision versus radical surgery. Many tumors below the anorectal line can be totally excised for cure, while those at the anorectal line usually require radical surgery. In my experience, a tumor near or encroaching on the anorectal line has a worse prognosis than one at the anal verge or perianal area. A tumor near the anorectal line has a threefold chance of metastasizing, superiorally by way of the superior hemorrhoidals, laterally by way of the middle hemorrhoidals, and to the inguinal nodes. There is a narrow zone of transitional epithelium at the dentate or anorectal line. Tumors arising in this area may have certain characteristics of the cells in this area, which accounts for the previously mentioned histologic variants of squamous cell carcinoma.

STAGING AND CLASSIFICATION OF CANCER

Introduction

Grading and classification are techniques for describing the extent of cancer that have significance in planning treatment for and estimating the prognosis of the disease. A widely accepted and useful classification of cancer according to microscopic and gross findings has yet to be devised. This is unfortunate because Broders and Dukes performed the necessary research

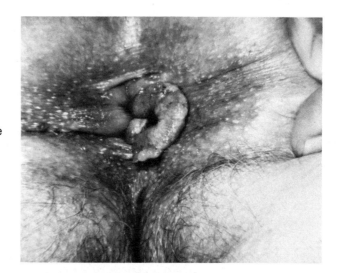

Figure 15–5. Adenocarcinoma of the rectum invading the anal canal.

and as pathologists had access to a vast amount of biopsy and surgical specimens. From their efforts evolved an almost perfect system of classification of colorectal cancer according to pathology. Broders' system of microscopic grading of tumors has yet to be improved upon. Dukes' classification has proved difficult to modify without confusing many physicians.

Although efforts to improve existing classifications are justifiable and useful, the end result could well be a system so complex and detailed that it will not be properly interpreted or generally accepted. Furthermore, any new system is subject to its own inherent errors of interpretation. For example, the new modifications of the Dukes method, which we use at our own hospital, attach the name Dukes A to a lesion limited to the mucosa. Such a cancer would not be invasive but rather carcinoma in situ. Dukes did not include noninvasive cancers in his classification, and one can readily understand how the five-year survival rates of the new studies are not easily compared with those of the earlier series.

Perhaps the TNM system, which is a clinical as well as pathologic classification, will prove to be the most useful. It is an extensive, sophisticated appraisal and survey of all phases of tumor and its extensions and metastases using the following parameters: primary tumor (T), regional lymph nodes (N), and distant metastases (M). Beahrs and Beart have written extensively concerning this innovation. The American Joint Committee for Cancer Staging and End Results Reporting has recommended a new TNM classification for colorectal cancers, as reported by Beart et al. in 1978.

Broders' Method of Grading

Broders first described the grading of cancer of the rectum (adenocarcinoma) according to histologic appearance in 1925. This was modified by Grinnell in 1939, and the Grinnell classification is generally now used, with several modifications.

The original Broders' classification represents in my opinion an excellent piece of basic research. All biopsy specimens were graded and when the surgical specimens, either polyps or segments of the rectum, became available, these were also graded and then correlated with the biopsy reports. Since various surgical pathologists performed the examinations, the research proved to be objective. In the majority of patients, the grading of the biopsy report and that of the surgical specimen proved to be identical. In only a few instances was there a considerable difference. Grade 1 adenocarcinoma showed slight differentiation in a glandular neoplasm similar to that seen in basal cell carcinoma of the skin. In Grade 2, the acini are not as well defined and the cells not as well differentiated as they are in a Grade 1 malignancy. In Grade 3 adenocarcinoma, the acini are ill defined and the nuclei irregular and large in proportion to the cytoplasm. In Grade 4 adenocarcinoma, there is very little tendency to form acini and practically all the cells are undifferentiated.

At one time various researchers described five grades of adenocarcinoma of the rectum, but they later revised this to correspond to Grinnell's classification, which comprises four categories: low-grade, average-grade, and high-grade malignancies, and mucoid carcinomas. All researchers subsequent to Broders included only invasive carcinomas. It might be well from a practical point of view and to avoid confusion to follow the suggestion of Bussey, who does not use numbers in his grading system but merely classifies them as low-grade, average-grade, and high-grade malignancies. In extensive studies, Bussey has found that the five-year survival rates are inversely proportional to the grade of malignancy.

Dukes' Classification

At the present time, the Dukes' staging procedure for cancer of the rectum is universally accepted throughout the world. When Dukes first described this procedure, he limited it to the rectum; however, it can also be applied to the colon. It is a simple although not perfect method of staging, and until the TNM system is accepted, I am certain that Dukes' classification will continue to be of value. Dukes' Stage A lesions extend below the basement membrane (muscularis mucosa), but not through the muscularis propria, bowel, or rectal wall. Dukes' Stage B lesions show invasion through the serosa or fascia propria of the rectum but without lymph node metastases. Stage C lesions show lymph node metastases regardless of depth of invasion: C_1 indicates paracolonic lymph node metastases only and C_2 indicates metastases in nodes up to the ligature of the large blood vessels. Dukes' Stage D lesions involve the liver or other distant metastases. On the basis of over 2000 cases of colorectal cancer, Morgan found 15 per cent to be Stage A, 35 per cent Stage B, and 50 per cent Stage C. The five-year survival rates for Dukes' classification are: Stage A, 98 per cent; Stage B, 78 per cent; Stage C, 32 per cent; and Stage D, 0 per cent. *Corman's statistics* show a slight improvement in survival rates.

The Dukes' staging procedure has been modified in order to be more accurate as to which layer of the bowel or rectum has been penetrated by cancer: stage A, Lesions limited to the mucosa; B, Lesions extending into the muscularis propria with negative nodes; B_2, lesions extending into pericolic fat with negative nodes; C_1, lesions limited to the bowel wall with positive nodes; C_2, lesions extending through all layers of the bowel wall with positive nodes; and D, lesions involving the liver or other distant metastases. This modification is used at the Sacred Heart Hospital, and closely follows the classification used at the Mayo Clinic, where it originated.

ETIOLOGY

The exact cause of colorectal cancer is unknown, although both the clinician and the researcher are aware of certain factors that may influence the development of colorectal cancer. These factors may be environmental, genetic, or certain colorectal diseases that may predispose to malignant tumors.

One can postulate that cancer occurs in a "diseased" colon. It is not limited to a colon harboring premalignant dysplastic conditions such as certain polyps or long-standing inflammatory bowel disease. If this is true, cancer can develop in "diseased" bodies in which host resistance is reduced. Immunologic or dietary deficiences would play a part in this process.

Environmental Factors

With the exception of Japan, colorectal cancer is more common in the countries that enjoy high economic development, such as the United States, where the diet tends to be high in fat and low in fiber. Colorectal cancer is less prevalent in those countries where a high-fiber, low-fat, and relatively low-protein diet is consumed. Goldberg and colleagues state that strict vegetarians have 40 per cent less colorectal cancer. In a recent study, they have shown that while dietary intake of animal fat and protein does not change the number or type of fecal microflora, it may change their metabolic activity. Dietary fat is known to increase bile acid degradation, which is believed to contribute to the formation of carcinogens. Our Western diet may favor a flora that may enzymatically metabolize acid and neutral steroids to carcinogens.

On the other hand, inhibition of carcinogenesis may occur by certain enzymes such as benzpyrene hydroxylase. There are certain foods, such as cabbage and cauliflower, which increase the activity of this enzyme. Wattenberg claims that certain antioxidants which are added to foods produce inhibition of experimental carcinogenesis. Various vitamins and minerals, such as vitamin C, vitamin A, and selenium, have also been proposed as potential inhibitors of the neoplastic process. An increased amount of dietary fiber may bind a greater proportion of bile salts and their metabolites, and increase their secretion. Another possibility is that fiber may dilute the potential carcinogen or at least safely "escort" it through the intestinal tract.

Genetic Factors

Although most colorectal cancers are believed to be due to environmental factors, there are certain heredity diseases that definitely predispose to colorectal cancer. Congenital multiple polyposis is one such disease. There are various fairly well-defined syndromes associated with this condition, the most common of which is Gardner's syndrome (see Chap. 13). The syndrome usually manifests itself with bloody diarrhea at puberty. The polyps are generally limited to the colon and rectum, and sometimes are associated with mesenchymal benign tumors such as fibromas of the abdominal wall or mesentery of the bowel, or osteomas of the jaw. If colectomy or proctocolectomy is not performed at the appropriate time most of these patients will develop colorectal cancer before 40 years of age.

Another syndrome associated with congenital multiple polyposis is Turcot's syndrome, which consists of polyps of the colon in association with tumors of the central nervous system. Peutz-Jeghers syndrome is characterized by pigment deposits in various parts of the body, particularly the lips, and by hamartomatous polyps of the gastrointestinal tract that carry no malignant potential.

Predisposition to Cancer

Inflammatory Bowel Disease. All authors agree that inflammatory bowel disease is a premalignant condition, especially if the entire colon is involved with onset at an early age, and if the disease has been of more than 10 years' duration. Every doctor treating more than an occasional patent with chronic ulcerative colitis will eventually see a high-grade cancer of the colon or rectum that is the direct result of long-standing disease. My own statistics indicate an overall rate of malignancy in 1 per cent of inflammatory bowel disease, including ulcerative proctitis. However, ulcerative colitis patients demonstrating involvement of the entire colon with a duration (from history given by patient) of 5 to 40 years revealed malignant degeneration in 4 per cent of cases. Ulcerative colitis limited to the left colon may also cause cancer but requires an additional 10 years. Crohn's disease, the other segment of inflammatory bowel disease, was not originally thought to be a precancerous lesion. However, in 1973, Weedon and Shorter showed that these patients are at considerable risk.

Evidence of epithelial dysplasia on rectal biopsy of ulcerative colitis has been viewed as a precancerous condition. Since the prognosis for advanced colitis carcinoma is poor, British workers have advocated prophylactic proctocolectomy in selected patients with biopsies positive for epithelial dysplasia. This would be a distinct advantage. American pathologists generally have not developed this skill to a degree comparable to those workers in England.

Waye summarized the problem and suggests the use of annual multiple biopsies for patients with universal ulcerative collitis who have had the disease at least 10 years. He lists other indications for colonoscopy other than surveillance, such as examination of a mass of stricture demonstrable by barium enema and as an aid in differentiating Crohn's disease from ulcerative colitis. While a narrow colon caused by strictures may impede a colonoscope, Waye often surmounts this difficulty by using a pediatric endoscope. He emphasizes the importance of the colonoscope in the search for atypia and carcinoma in situ and views colonoscopy as an adjunct to rather than a replacement for barium enema.

Polyps. Between 6 and 12 per cent of people are found to have either sessile or pedunculated polyps in the colon or rectum. They vary in size from a few millimeters to several centimeters in diameter. Villous polyps can carpet almost the entire mucosa of the rectum.

Polyps are considered premalignant lesions. No one completely understands the polyp-cancer sequence. Of course, a polyp should be excised or fulgurated, but one containing a nidus of malignancy without involvement of its stalk does not require a cancer resection.

DIAGNOSIS

In colorectal cancer, especially rectal cancer where a colostomy might be a consideration, it is especially important to be accurate in the diagnosis. The pathologist's diagnosis of carcinoma in situ may not really mean cancer. According to many specialists, particularly the group from St. Mark's Hospital in London, when there is no invasion of the basement membrane (muscularis mucosa), there is no malignancy. The only cancer that has real significance is invasive cancer, the type that may require radical surgery. Any pathologist will readily admit that it is difficult to make a diagnosis from the small amount of tissue submitted following biopsy. In fact, in some cases the entire lesion must be submitted before the presence or absence of invasion can be determined. In deciding on treatment, especially when sacrifice of the rectum is involved, the surgeon should rely on gross characteristics of the lesion as well as the laboratory report.

In a complex disease such as cancer, a "second look" or a second opinion by the same surgeon is important. In difficult decisions, I frequently ask myself, "What would I want done if I were the patient"? I mention this to demonstrate how difficult it is to diagnose cancer without considering the diagnosis of premalignant lesions or even the lesions associated with cancer both within and outside the colon.

Usually, when a diagnosis of colorectal cancer is made and a complete colonoscopic examination is conducted, there will be gross polyps or at least mamillations found in other parts of the colon. In fact, 3 to 4 per cent of such patients will demonstrate one or more additional cancers.

ESTABLISHING PATIENT CONFIDENCE

Every patient who comes to the office, regardless of age or complaints, should be considered a potential cancer patient. In my practice, I prefer to make a general statement at the beginning of the examination, such as, "Let's look you over from A to Z. The chances are we'll find nothing seriously wrong, but you will feel better knowing this fact." The actual examination can be taken a step at a time. I deliberately avoid mentioning the word "cancer" because even the simplest examination can be an ordeal if performed on an apprehensive patient. The patient is an emotional being and acts, behaves, and makes decisions accordingly. It is best to examine and treat patients with this in mind and to utilize every bit of knowledge available to help the patient relax. One must exude confidence and reassurance. Everything a physician says or does must be done gently. A trusting, relaxed patient will tolerate even painful procedures without a complaint.

HISTORY

A good history is worth the effort. It is important to note diet, bowel habits, and the past medical and family history, especially as it relates to cancer and precancerous conditions such as congenital multiple polyposis and colitis. An experienced secretary or nurse can obtain most of this information before the actual consultation.

I frequently ask the patient what they think is wrong. In this manner, many previously hidden clues or inner fears will be exposed. I will ask the patient to "feed everything into the computer." I ask for the chief complaint first. In my experience this is usually bleeding. Jackman states that practically all cancers of the bowel will bleed and I agree, although a Hemoccult test may be necessary to prove it. It is important to know the amount and color, whether or not it is mixed with the stool, whether it occurs only at stool, and over what period of time it has been occurring. Also important to know is whether the amount is increasing and whether it is seen only in the stool or on the underwear or also when straining at stool. Some will say the bleeding occurs also when expelling flatus. Others will state that they hear blood drip into the toilet bowl when they first bear down on bowel movement.

Bleeding from cancer of the colon and rectum is usually mixed with the stool. Cancers of the anal area and the lower rectum additionally produce the so-called surface bleeding seen on the tissue and underwear. The character of the bleeding in colorectal cancer depends on the location of the tumor. The color varies from red to maroon and even black, depending on whether the tumor is at the anorectal area or cecum. Transit time of the stool may also control color. Patients with cecal cancer may pass red blood in the stools or actual diarrhea. By the same token, the dark-red to black blood seen in some patients with cecal cancer may be due to constipation,which allows the blood to undergo autolysis and other physiologic changes.

In developing more information concerning the bleeding, it is important to know what other symptoms are associated with it, such as pain at the anus, protrusion, diarrhea, abdominal cramps, constipation, upper gastrointestinal problems, esophageal symptoms, cardiovascular problems, or rectal tenesmus. Many patients complain of abdominal pain. Usually abdominal pain is a late symptom and occurs when the tumor has grown sufficiently to cause some degree of obstruction. Tumors of the rectum, and particularly in the lower rectum, are apt to produce the urge to defecate or tenesmus. This is in direct proportion to the size of the tumor and its proximity to the anus. Sometimes the patient goes to the toilet and merely attempts to defecate or expels only flatus or bloody mucus. Fecal impaction can produce similar symptoms, including bloody mucus, and can easily be diagnosed by digital examination. In fact, fecal impactions higher in the colon are frequently confused with tumors at barium enema examinations. As with other diagnostic problems, colonoscopy can quickly confirm the diagnosis. Other conditions causing rectal tenesmus are inflammatory bowel disease, foreign bodies, and irritating enemas.

EXTERNAL INSPECTION

Most patients will have had a thorough physical examination before coming to your office, and a general physical is not always necessary or feasible. An examination of the abdomen and groin is important, however. One must always look for distention due to obstruction. Inguinal nodes must be examined for metastases.

DIGITAL EXAMINATION

The "educated" index finger is the most important instrument at the surgeon's command. It alone, of all methods, can examine almost all of the pelvis. Its field is not limited to the anal canal and rectum but encompasses almost all structures from the sacrum to the pubic area.

A digital examination can diagnose at least 35 per cent of colorectal cancers. Furthermore, it can diagnose most pelvic abscesses due to perforating cancers or diverticulitis of the sigmoid. It is useful too in diagnosing some cases of appendicitis and diverticulitis of the cecum. As an aid in differential diagnosis, the index finger is almost unbelievable.

With the tip of the finger at the rectosigmoid, which is not impossible in slender individuals, the patient is asked to bear down. Occasionally a sigmoidal cancer may be palpated in this manner. There is nothing that feels quite like a cancer. It is stony hard. The tumor's extent, resectability, and attachment to other structures can largely be determined by the digital examination. It is possible to palpate masses in the rectouterine or retrovesical pouch such as the hard, fixed shelflike projection known as Blumer's shelf, which is due to metastases from a cancer higher in the abdomen. Although this can be due to bleeding at the anus, blood on the examining finger is significant. Stool on the finger can be used for a Hemoccult test.

INSTRUMENTATION

After digital examination and providing there are no contraindications, a proctosigmoidoscopic examination can be conducted. The trauma from even a carefully conducted examination can easily convert a walled-off pelvic abscess into peritonitis or an acute diverticulitis into a perforation. Contraindications for this examination include an acute abdomen or acute fulminating colitis. In these cases, proctoscopic examination should suffice.

Proctosigmoidoscopy can rule out at least 60 per cent of colorectal cancers, and if bloody mucus or stool is seen, it may suggest the presence of a bleeding lesion higher in the colon. If a raised, ulcerating cauliflower-like lesion is seen, biopsy can be performed, taking a small bite of tissue from the friable lesion itself and not near the area where it is attached to normal bowel. If this precaution is not exercised, stubborn and sometimes serious bleeding may result. Cancerous tissue is like very hard cheese and does not require a sharp biopsy; normal tissue is elastic and easily movable. For these reasons, I use the Buie biopsy forceps, which will not easily injure normal tissue except by tugging or tearing by the operator. I frequently test the tissue first, making sure that the tissue grasped is cancerous, before taking the bite.

The technique of colonoscopy has been discussed in Chapter 3. Colonoscopic and x-ray examinations of the colon must supplement each other. There are times when colonoscopy cannot be performed due to adhesions from previous surgery, anatomic variations of the colon, or extreme spasm. Rarely, small cancers will not be visualized on colonoscopy but will be detected by the double-contrast barium enema.

PLAIN X-RAY EXAMINATION

It would be difficult to diagnose colon disease without the aid of the flat plate of the abdomen and the barium enema. In fact, when the history and examination indicate that flatus and/or stool is not being passed or that there is distention and/or tenderness anywhere in the abdomen, the flat plate or obstructive x-ray series is the first test to be ordered. The x-ray of the abdomen should precede the proctosigmoidoscopic examination because the air that enters the lower bowel during proctosigmoidoscopy may make proper interpretation of the plain film more difficult.

Obstruction. With obvious exceptions such as volvulus and a cecum that is distended to a diameter of 9 cm or more, there is no urgency associated with the diagnosis of colon obstruction as there is with small bowel obstruction. High-grade small bowel obstruction with sudden onset of vomiting, abdominal distention with pain, inability to pass gas and stool, tenderness, and audible peristalsis, and with x-ray showing a loop of distended bowel presents no real problem in diagnosis and treatment. Generalized paralytic ileus with vomiting, abdominal distention, inability to pass gas and stool, very little pain or tenderness, absent bowel sounds, soft abdomen, and x-ray demonstrating gaseous distention of both small and large bowel also provides little difficulty in diagnosis and treatment, especially if it occurs in the hospital following major surgery.

However, small bowel obstruction can evade the most carefully performed clinical examination and laboratory aids available, including x-ray examination. Laboratory tests can actually be misleading. For instance, the white blood count and flat plate of the abdomen may be normal in early obstruction and strangulation, or the white blood count may be high in dehydration with no strangulation.

The grey zone between these extremes of obvious obstruction and suggestive but inconclusive evidence is what really concerns the physician in the diagnosis of obstructing or perforating cancer. In interpreting the plain film of the abdomen one must keep in mind the following facts: high obstructions in the duodenum or upper jejunum may produce no positive x-ray signs on flat plate. Even the stomach may be empty due to vomiting. The character and onset of the vomiting depend on the location of the obstruction. It may require hours for the onset of fecal vomiting from obstruction of the lower small intestine and days for this sign to develop in colon obstruction if the ileocecal valve is incompetent. If this valve is competent, in some cases of colon obstruction it is possible for the cecum to perforate without vomiting. When the colon is obstructed and the ileocecal valve is incompetent, the gas and feces may accumulate first in the colon and then the overflow will back up into the small intestine. In fact, if the obstruction is at the ileocecal area, there may be no gas or stool in the colon and the x-ray findings would be due to distention of the small bowel.

The radiologist and clinician must work together to make difficult diagnoses and must constantly keep the normal anatomy in mind. The radiologist can only determine the presence or absence of flatus, fecal material, or a combination of both that produces the air-fluid levels. Air-fluid levels may be found in normal individuals following enemas; however, the water runs into the small bowel only if the ileocecal valve is incompetent.

Radiologic examination can be of great help in diagnosing a large bowel obstruction. A dilated colon above the area of obstruction is usually seen on plain film x-ray of the abdomen. Obstructing cancers of the colon usually occur in the left colon from the splenic flexure to the rectosigmoid. If after sigmoidoscopic and x-ray examination there is still doubt as to whether the partial or complete obstruction is in the large or small bowel, or if there is doubt as to the approximate location of the obstruction in the colon, a barium enema should be ordered. Even though the barium goes in a retrograde fashion through the obstructed area, it is not wise to continue introducing more barium after the diagnosis is made, since the barium may precipitate a complete obstruction or may be difficult to remove. This occasionally occurs in spite of all the modern technical advances in radiology. In the absence of perforation of the bowel, this factor is of less importance in the small bowel than in the colon. The succus entericus in the small bowel dilutes the barium, making it relatively easy to retrieve. It is interesting to note that obstruction from the retrograde flow of barium does not always mean that the colon is completely occluded or that flatus and/or stool cannot pass downward in the regular way.

Although x-ray remains the best diagnostic aid in bowel obstruction, I have found, as Welch pointed out, that air rises quickly in the intestinal tract and therefore, on x-ray of the abdomen, air may not be found directly above or at the area of obstruction. This is particularly true in the small bowel, where air may be found by x-ray to be many feet above or proximal to the obstruction.

Possible Perforation. In my experience, aside from cecal perforations, free perforations into the peritoneal cavity are relatively rare. The presence of an acute abdomen with or without x-ray confirmation requires immediate surgery.

In Greenbaum's *Radiographic Atlas of Colon Disease,* Novy describes diastatic rupture of the cecum. The muscle separates first by the bulging mucosa, which eventually perforates. Given equal pressure throughout the colon the greatest distention occurs in that portion of the colon with the greatest diameter, the cecum. The law of Laplace, which states that the pressure required to distend the walls of a hollow viscus is inversely proportional to its radius, applies in this case.

A colorectal cancer that perforates usually is an advanced lesion and generally occurs in an individual who has had colicky abdominal pains on and off for some months. It is usually accompained by complete or partial obstruction indicated by difficulty or inability to pass flatus and/or stool. Abdominal distention, fever, and all the other signs of abscess accompany this condition. Depending on the stage of this complication, there may be signs of localized peritoneal irritation with a mass. The abscess may be sealed off by the abdominal wall or another portion of intestine or by another organ such as the small bowel, bladder, or stomach. This is more common in the lower sigmoid but may occur anywhere in the colon.

BARIUM ENEMA EXAMINATION

The barium enema examination should be considered a valuable aid in the diagnosis of colon disease. I am amazed at the number of small cancers and polyps that the radiologist is able to detect in the colon and even the rectum. Although the rectum is not the usual area for diagnosis using the indirect method of double contrast barium enema, I have occasionally been surprised by the radiologist's report of a rectal polyp after I had performed the usual proctosigmoidoscopic examination. Barium enema examination has limitations, however. Some claim that 9 per cent of cancers are missed on the initial examination. Poor preparation has been cited as the cause for this relatively high failure rate. Thus, as previously noted, barium enema and colonoscopy should be considered complementary procedures, establishing the primary diagnosis. Ultrasonography and computed tomography (CT) are used in helping to delineate extensions and recurrences of neoplasms.

Indications. With the high incidence of cancer and precancerous lesions in the Western world, it is important that everyone past 40 years of age without symptoms have an x-ray or colonoscopic examination of the cecum every two to three years. Those with symptoms suggesting cancer or with a positive Hemoccult test should have an x-ray examination regardless of age. For younger people, patients with considerable x-ray exposure, and those not wishing to have x-ray, I do not hesitate to suggest colonoscopy.

Contraindications. The absolute contraindications for barium enema examination are toxic megacolon and free perforations. In suspected walled-off perforations with abscess formation, barium enema must be used with caution or not at all and only after consultation with the radiologist. There is always the danger of causing a free perforation or extending an area of limited peritonitis. Rigler reported a mortality rate of 51 per cent in 50 patients with free perforations due to barium. The prognosis is better if immediate surgery is performed. A small amount of barium to demonstrate an abscess or fistula to the bladder or vagina, however, does no harm. Barium in the general peritoneal cavity must be removed as quickly as possible. It is difficult to evacuate, but it is an irritant and will eventually cause peritonitis and adhesions.

Interpretation. Diagnostic radiology should properly be left to the radiologist. However, there are certain reasons for the clinician to review all films and allow the patient to do so also, whether or not abnormalities are found. The clinician will learn something about diagnostic radiology and its limitations, and the patient will be pleased by the interest shown. Occasionally, in this manner, a lesion or suspected lesion will be found that was not previously seen. The variations of the normal colon will be appreciated, and the need for colonoscopic examination determined. Radiologic examination of the colon is not an exact science, and for a definitive diagnosis, colonoscopic examination is frequently suggested by the radiologist. When colonoscopy is not feasible, the surgeon must see all appropriate films when selecting the optimum area for incision.

A knowledge of the pathology of cancerous and precancerous lesions will help ensure better interpretation of x-rays. Practically all cancers of the colon are adenocarcinomas, and most of these are the ulcerating type. Unfortunately, some are small with very little if any elevation above the mucosal surface. In these cases one looks for mucosal destruction. If there is reasonable doubt, it is mandatory to resort to colonoscopy. There is very little problem if the lesion is large, especially when it is annular and presents the typical apple-core deformity on x-ray examination.

Polypoid cancer, the next most frequent adenocarcinoma of the colon, also varies in size, usually has a wide base, grows toward the lumen of the bowel, and is therefore higher than the ulcerating type. It more frequently occurs in the right colon. It may be confused with a polyp, since as it enlarges the mucosa becomes elevated and creates the false impression of having a pedicle. This is known as a pseudopedunculated lesion. Scirrhous cancer is irregular and involves a greater length of colon than the other types. It tends to occur in older individuals and in the left colon.

Lymphosarcoma is frequently part of a generalized disease. It has a predilection for the ileocecal area but may occur anywhere in the bowel. It has no pathognomonic radiologic signs, and although it usually involves larger segments of the colon than adenocarcinoma, it may occasionally have a "napkin-ring" appearance. Leiomyoma and leiomyosarcoma present as intramural diseases, since they are tumors of smooth muscle. They are firm tumors, and although the overlying mucosa is usually normal, they may be seen as they intrude on the bowel lumen.

Differential Diagnosis. The clinician is not expected to become a radiologist, but he should be concerned with the differential diagnosis of common colorectal diseases. Fortunately, this is easy with modern x-ray technics, except in certain diseases. The inflammatory feature of diverticulitis may make it difficult to rule out a hidden carcinoma that may be too small for visualization. Furthermore, larger cancers may produce x-ray findings similar to that of diverticulitis. However, repeat x-rays are frowned upon by many patients and physicians because of the possible radiation effects. Furthermore, the bowel may be so narrow that even endoscopy, except with a special narrow or pediatric-size endoscope, may be difficult. Cytologic examination of colon washings for neoplastic cells may have a definite use here.

Intramural or submucosal tumors such as simple lipomas may defy accurate diagnosis without laparotomy. Extrinsic tumors such as endometrioma and cancer implants shown by x-ray as indefinite defects need clinical correlation. The mucosal pattern is normal but there is evidence of extrinsic pressure on the colon.

The clinician who sees a lot of colon and rectal disease is constantly faced with x-rays showing benign defects. These could be due to a prominent ileocecal valve, lipomatous hypertrophy of the ileocecal valve, inverted appendiceal stumps, polyps, particles of stool, bubbles of air, or simply artefacts that must be ruled out by endoscopy. If endoscopy is not possible, repeat x-rays are often helpful. If doubt still exists, exploratory laparotomy is justified.

Strictures due to inflammatory bowel disease are worrisome to both the radiologist and the clinician. Representative specimens at biopsy and endoscopy are difficult to obtain. Therefore, strictures, unless proven soft and pliable with negative biopsy report, may be another indication for justifiable laparotomy. The general approach for the clinician, as far as differential x-ray diagnosis is concerned, is to attempt diagnosis of the common problem and to place the rare ones in a separate group labeled "abnormal with etiology undetermined" and leave this group for interpretation by the radiologist.

LAPAROSCOPY

Laparoscopy may help in diagnosing metastatic disease and in differentiating endometriosis and other pelvic disease from cancer of the colon. There certainly is a risk of perforating the colon in metastatic disease because the bowel tends to be fixed and matted together, and the disease is seldom limited to the cul-de-sac or ovaries.

CLOSED-NEEDLE BIOPSY OF THE LIVER

In diagnosis of metastatic disease of the colon, this procedure is extremely limited unless the liver is massively involved, enlarged, and palpable. A negative result means nothing, and there is always the danger of hemorrhage from the procedure.

CYTOLOGIC EXAMINATION

Raskin first described this method of examining centrifuged specimens obtained from washings of the colon. The method proved to be too involved and time-consuming, and has generally been replaced by endoscopy. It may still have an extremely limited use in differentiating cancer from diverticulitis if endoscopy is not possible.

TREATMENT

General Principles

For the average patient with colorectal cancer, preparation for surgery begins in the office. A detailed discussion with the physician tends to establish confidence on the part of the patient. The greatest fear the patient has is that of cancer. There are some patients who will become depressed and uncooperative upon being told they have cancer. Good judgment will serve to identify this type of patient. The family or one particular family member must know the facts. Some patients will be relieved to know that they have a low grade of cancer, which is often true in rectal cancer, and acceptance becomes somewhat easier.

The second greatest fear for the patient is that of possible establishment of a colostomy. If the cancer is in the colon or if it is possible to perform a sphincter-preserving operation, it should be easy to reassure the patient on this point. If the operation will definitely include colostomy, the patient should be told that with modern care of stomas this is a relatively small price to pay for a chance at cure. The enterostomal therapist can be of great help after the patient is admitted to the hospital.

The patient should be in a good psychologic and physiologic condition before entering the hospital. When the psychologic preparation for surgery is completed, the patient should be told about the importance of good nutrition and avoiding smoking, if relevant. Very few of my patients require hyperalimentation or exhausting tests while in the hospital. Most tests, x-ray studies, and colonoscopic examinations have been performed prior to admission. Except for a routine medical work-up and I.V. urogram, there are few tests performed in the hospital. Admission to the hospital one or two days prior to surgery is usually sufficient, except where there are medical problems requiring specific tests or preparations such as a brain scan or insertion of an artificial pacemaker.

I find that a short preparation, usually two days in length, will not disturb normal physiology. It consists of clear liquids by mouth and mechanical preparation of the bowel with one or two doses of 2 oz of castor oil by mouth and administration of water enemas until the fluid is absolutely clear. It is essential that the castor oil is effective. The surgeon or resident must question the patient on this point because this is the essential step in successful bowel surgery.

The patient is told about the importance of frequent deep breaths and coughing before surgery. The inhalation therapy service can be of great help. Leg exercises and frequent change in posture is encouraged after surgery. This instruction is important in preventing pneumonia, vascular problems, and other complications. It is essential to ambulate the patient beginning on the first day after surgery.

Both aerobic and anaerobic bacteria can be controlled by a short antibiotic preparation with neomycin and erythromycin. However, a sterile bowel is not desirable or safe because of the danger of enteritis. No amounts of antibiotics will prevent disruption of a suture line or other complications due to poor technic.

Surgical Management

With certain exceptions to be discussed later, adequate surgery is the only hope we have now or in the immediate future for complete cure of colorectal cancer. All other methods, including fulguration, chemotherapy, radiotherapy, and immunotherapy, must be considered as investigative. Such treatment, whether it be primary or adjuvant, should not be discouraged but should be controlled by well-organized, highly motivated cancer centers.

The rectum, which extends from the anorectal line to the rectosigmoid and measures approximately 16 cm in length, presents some interesting situations in dealing with cancer in this area of the colon. One must remember that 16 cm is a direct line measured with the sigmoidoscope from the anus to the rectosigmoid and that the rectum actually has two curves. Anteriorly and posteriorly, the rectum has the general contour of a bow, which allows the rectum to fit snugly in the hollow of the sacrum. Laterally, the rectum presents as an "S"-shaped curve. From a practical viewpoint, it is helpful to think of the rectum as divided into an upper half and a lower half, with the mid-portion of the rectum corresponding closely to the peritoneal reflection. Because the lymphatic, blood, and nerve supplies are different in the two halves of the rectum and because the rectum can be straightened after it is dissected free from the wall of the sacrum and from the lateral ligaments, sphincter-saving operations with anastomosis are logical and safe procedures.

The location of the growth largely determines the suitability of a lesion for a sphincter-saving operation. Lesions just above the dentate line will require an abdominoperineal resection, but for lesions higher in the rectum the decision will be made at the time of surgery, and the patient should be informed when this is the case. In most instances when the cancer is located in the upper half of the rectum, it is possible to do a sphincter-saving operation, either a low anterior resection or a pull-through procedure. A lesion in the lower portion of the rectum, especially one that is easily palpable with the finger, usually requires a Miles abdominoperineal resection. Of course, there are exceptions to every rule, and in some cases of early small cancers, I might perform a pull-through procedure or a low anterior resection for lesions extending to within 6 cm of the anus.

Cancers in the lower half of the rectum have a poor prognosis because the lymph channels allow for lateral as well as superior spread. The lymphatics also intermingle with the lymphatics of the posterior wall of the vagina; for that reason, the posterior wall of the vagina is frequently removed in the course of an abdominoperineal resection. Cancers in the upper half of the rectum have a superior lymphatic drainage only; therefore, their prognosis is much better. It is also feasible to do a primary anastomosis for lesions in this area. If an anastomosis is not possible, either hand sewn, or with the stapler, a pull-through operation can be performed.

It is advisable to examine the cancer very carefully before surgery, not only with the finger but with the sigmoidoscope or anoscope if necessary. Sometimes on digital examination the lesion seems to be fixed and inoperable, when at operation it is easily removable. I am particularly careful during examination to determine if the cancer involves the prostate or bladder. Urograms, cystoscopic examinations, and other tests, which may include the CT scan, are required. The rest of the colon should be examined by x-ray or colonoscopic examination or both to rule out additional lesions in other areas of the colon. If colostomy is anticipated, the site for the stoma is marked by the enterostomal therapist the day before surgery. Any stoma which is not brought out through the midline or one of the rectus muscles will be accompanied by a parastomal bulge or hernia (Figs. 15–6 to 15–8).

The abdomen is explored carefully, including the entire small bowel. The tumor may have extended to the cervix, uterus, small bowel, appendix, or bladder and this must be determined at this time. Hysterectomy or removal of portions of the bladder or small bowel is frequently necessary. The matter of grossly normal ovaries, which in 4 per cent of cases harbor metastatic malignancy or even a primary malignancy of the ovary, has not fully been evaluated, although recently I have been performing excision of tubes and ovaries in practically all cancers in the upper rectum. I do this even in the premenstrual patient on the basis of Ferguson's work. If there is a solitary,

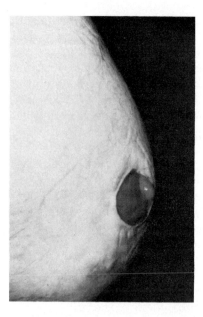

Figure 15–6. Parastomal hernia.

accessible metastasis in the liver that has proved to be cancerous by frozen section, that portion of the liver is removed. I have no personal experience with complete lobectomies and believe that this type of treatment is investigational at the present time. Patients requiring this type of surgery are referred to surgeons with special expertise in this area.

Naturally in rectal cancers, it is impossible to use surgical tapes above and below the lesion, although a cancer in the upper portion of the rectum after it is mobilized can be treated in this manner. In surgery for cancer of the rectum, it is relatively easy to ligate the inferior mesenteric vessels at their origin early in the operation, thus permitting a wider and easier dissection. If I do not have enough viable bowel for anastomosis if an anastomotic procedure is considered expedient, I do not hesitate to mobilize the splenic flexure. There are exceptions to ligating the inferior mesenteric vessels at their origin, for example, a markedly obese patient or one in which a resection is deemed palliative. High ligation does not increase the cure rate but provides added length to the bowel when this is desirable. A decision as

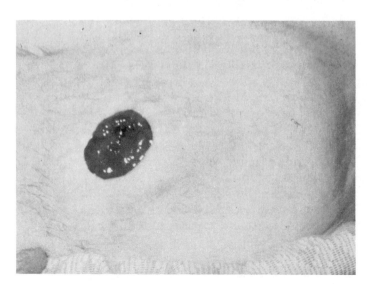

Figure 15–7. Properly placed colonic stoma.

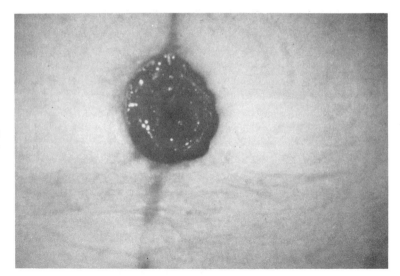

Figure 15–8. Stoma brought out through midline incision.

to the type of operation necessary is not made until the rectum is well mobilized down to the levators, which means that the rectum is free from the prostate and from the hollow of the sacrum down to the tip of the coccyx. One need not worry about the blood supply to the stump of the rectum. In my entire experience, I have never seen a slough due to lack of blood supply to the distal segment of rectum. If anastomosis is anticipated, one must be sure to be well below the tumor, approximately 5 cm is ideal. The pull-through operation is a highly selective and still controversial procedure. To put it simply, I utilize the pull-through operation when a lesion is too high to sacrifice the sphincters and too low to perform a satisfactory anastomosis. I consider the pull-through procedure at the present time to be a compromise. I learned early that sloughs following the pull-through procedure are due to reliance on the marginal artery of Drummond for revascularization. Furthermore, thrombosis of the marginal artery of Drummond can produce complications. For this reason, when I perform a pull-through procedure, I modify the operation by not taking the vessels at their origin. I ligate the sigmoidal vessels individually and like to see a little mesentery on the bowel to be pulled through.

MILES ABDOMINOPERINEAL RESECTION

In recent years, a low midline incision has been used that can be curved around and above the umbilicus when necessary. High ligation of the inferior mesenteric vessels is performed early, but it is not done flush with the aorta in obese patients and those who undergo palliative resections. Grinnell's findings indicate that when the highest of the inferior mesenteric lymph nodes are involved, the malignant cells usually have spread beyond the reach of a radical operation. High ligation should include the left colic artery, and sometimes this may be important in evaluating the blood supply to the portion of the bowel that is used for the colonic stoma. Pelvic lymphadenectomy is not routinely performed, since it merely prolongs the operation and appears to increase the likelihood of immediate and late complications. Occasionally, the uterus, the posterior wall of the vagina, a portion of involved bladder, the appendix, or a portion of the small bowel is removed. In suitable cases, if the liver is involved, a wedge resection may be performed. The internal iliac arteries are not ligated routinely, because this step does not seem to lessen blood loss significantly.

The colostomy is established through a separate stab wound. The day before the operation a suitable site is chosen by the enterostomal therapist. It is not necessary to close the paracolic gutter. The stoma is left open and its margins sutured to the skin edge.

Although it may be considered desirable to clamp and ligate the lateral ligaments with their associated arteries, it is usually not necessary. These ligaments and arteries can be cut easily with a scissors, and there is seldom any bleeding.

The perineal phase of the operation is performed with the patient in the lithotomy position. It is not necessary to remove the coccyx. During this phase of the operation, occasionally one cuts through tumor tissue that appears to be attached to the pelvic wall, the prostatic capsule, or the tissues adjacent to the membranous urethra. While a zealous attempt is made to remove all of the diseased tissue without invading normal structures (Fig. 15–9), sometimes one has to cut into the rectum. Undoubtedly, there are occasions when cancer cells escape, despite irrigations and other available preventive measures. After the operation is completed, a large gauze pack is introduced. It is removed on the sixth or seventh day, and usually the patient can be discharged on the tenth to twelfth day after operation. If adequate extirpation is performed, closure of the posterior wound is simply not feasible. Mere closure of the skin is not a true closure and there is no advantage.

In a group of 100 consecutive patients on whom I performed Miles' abdominoperineal resections, 14 had Dukes' Stage A lesions, 36 had Dukes' Stage B lesions, and 50 had Dukes' Stage C lesions. The five-year survival rate was 41.6 per cent. In a group of 209 consecutive Miles' resections, the operative mortality was 1.9 per cent.

LOW ANTERIOR RESECTION

The abdominal dissection is similar to that used in the Miles' operation, except that the rectum is transected well below the lesion. A suitable area of the sigmoid colon is also transected and the specimen removed (Fig. 15–10).

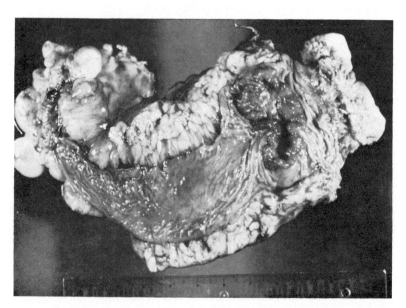

Figure 15–9. Surgical specimen obtained at abdominoperineal resection.

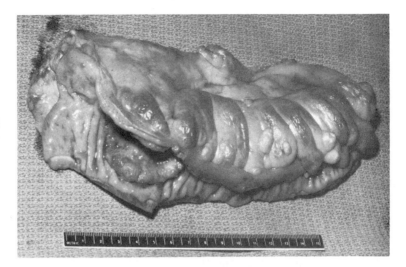

Figure 15–10. Specimen obtained from anterior resection.

A single-layer anastomosis is performed. If necessary, the posterior layer of sutures can be placed before tying the knots. Each suture must include the full thickness of the bowel wall. The posterior row is tied inside the lumen, and then, starting with an angle stitch, the anterior row of inverting sutures is placed and tied outside the lumen. The E.E.A. stapler is used occasionally when hand-sewn anastomoses are technically not possible. It is not necessary or desirable to close the peritoneal floor. A plastic sump drain is placed in the hollow of the sacrum and brought out through a separate stab wound. Two Penrose drains are placed, one in the pelvis and the other in the lateral gutter. The sump drain is attached to low suction and usually may be removed in one or two days. The other drains are removed gradually as indicated. The abdominal wall is closed with interrupted wire or polypropylene (Prolene) sutures, and the skin is closed in a similar fashion. Narrow Telfa strips are inserted at 2-inch intervals between the skin sutures down to the anterior fascia and are removed in several days. With the use of Telfa wicks, the incidence of wound infection is practically nil. A Levin nasogastric tube and Foley urinary catheter are used as indicated. Patients are usually ready for discharge on the tenth day after operation.

The five-year survival rate for a group of 113 consecutive low anterior resections was 58 per cent.

PULL-THROUGH PROCEDURE

Not all patients are suitable candidates for a safe pull-through operation. A patient selected for this procedure should have a long sigmoid colon. The procedure is currently performed through a low midline abdominal incision that extends a few inches above the umbilicus. It is now safer and more desirable to ligate the inferior mesenteric artery just below the left colic artery rather than at its origin. The marginal artery of Drummond provides a sufficient blood supply to at least the level of the mid-sigmoid. The mesentery below this point is removed with the specimen.

A pull-through operation should be performed only when viable sigmoid can be brought down easily to the tip of the coccyx. The entire rectum must be mobilized down to the levators. A sump drain placed in the hollow of the sacrum is brought out through a separate stab wound. The drain is usually removed within a few days. It is not necessary and usually not possible to

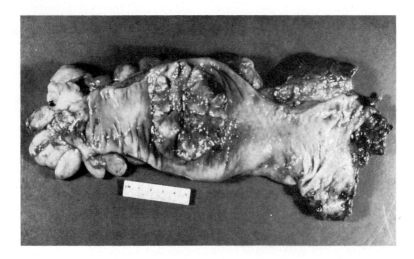

Figure 15–11. Specimen from pull-through operation.

close the peritoneal floor. After the abdomen has been closed, the patient is placed in the lithotomy position. The anus is dilated and the portion of rectum not freed previously is dissected from the sphincter mechanism, allowing as much anoderm to remain as possible. The levators are not disturbed. One must boldly dissect the anorectal segment from the levator muscles until the rectum is free of all remaining attachments to levators and prostate or vagina, as the case may be. More recently, I have not closed the abdomen until the perineal portion of the operation is completed. This is to avoid entrapment of the small bowel in the pelvis.

The rectum and sigmoid must be gently pulled through the denuded anal canal. The segment containing the tumor is transected after umbilical tape tie has been placed approximately 7 cm from the anus (Fig. 15–11). Gauze dressings are applied. The tape is removed after two days.

On the eighth postoperative day, simple anoplasty is performed, using local anesthesia. Postoperative care is similar to that following any anorectal operation. Patients are discharged on approximately the tenth postoperative day.

Survival rates for 120 consecutive patients undergoing pull-through procedures showed a 5-year survival rate of 49 per cent and a 20-year survival rate of 6 per cent. All survival rates are absolute, in that deaths from all causes are included.

Fulguration for Rectal Carcinoma

The overall 5-year survival rates for carcinoma of the lower third of the rectum are notoriously poor. In a group of 100 patients on whom I have performed the abdominoperineal resection for cancer of the lower rectum, the absolute survival rate was 41 per cent. Strauss was the first to suggest fulguration for rectal cancer. Madden, Turnbull, and Salvati and Rubin, have reported excellent 5-year survival rates for fulguration for certain cancers in the lower half of the rectum. The use of fulguration in the treatment of rectal cancer is a controversial issue, however, with most agreeing only that it has a use in the patient who is medically unfit for major surgery or who refuses surgery.

In my view, fulguration has a place in the treatment of cancer of the rectum, but it is not frequently used because most growths are not discovered early enough. I believe one indication for fulguration is an early freely movable cancer, preferably situated in the lower posterior portion of the rectum. In fact, I reported on 27 frank invasive cancers with an average distance of 8.8 cm above the dentate line and an average diameter of 2.81 cm. These were early, small, highly selected ulcerating invasive cancers. I admitted a number of these patients to the hospital for fulguration in one stage under spinal anesthesia. However, because of the high rate of secondary bleeding, I treated the others in the office by fractional fulguration without anesthesia. Only one of my office patients had a secondary hemorrhage. The average number of fulgurations in the 27 cases was 12.4. The lesion is gradually melted down at weekly intervals using light fulguration, until nothing but a raw surface or scar remains. If on two successive visits the tumor does not decrease in size and biopsy is positive, surgery must be considered.

The absolute 5-year survival rate in this group of patients proved to be 63.1 per cent. It should be emphasized that this series represented a highly selected group of early small cancers and that many years were required to accumulate this series of cases. I am not advocating office treatment for cancer. More recently, I have begun fulguration of large cancers in the hospital. Only patients with movable lesions located in the lower third of the rectum without palpable lymph nodes are selected. The Salvati method of fulguration of the full thickness of rectal wall, including a border of 1 cm of normal tissue, is used. Annular lesions involving the entire circumference of rectal wall are not suitable for fulguration because of the possibility of prolonged bleeding and stricture.

Treatment of Anorectal Cancer

SQUAMOUS CELL CARCINOMA

The synonyms for squamous cell carcinoma are epithelioma and epidermoid carcinoma. When they involve the skin of the perianal area or the lower part of the anal canal, the tumors behave as a squamous cell carcinoma occurring elsewhere in the body. The diagnosis must be confirmed by biopsy. Most tumors can be cured by local excision even if some of the sphincter muscle is involved. Selection for local excision depends on the location, which must be well away from the anorectal line, and the absence of deep penetration into the underlying muscle. There must be ample margin of at least 2 to 3 cm of normal tissue around the tumor. This is easy to obtain as far as the skin is concerned, but it is more difficult to remove this much tissue when muscle is involved without a certain degree of incontinence. This is a risk the patient must assume. Furthermore, in patients with short anal canals it may be difficult to obtain sufficient normal margin without extending the excision above the anorectal line and removing a portion of the mucosa.

I do not consider patients with early cancers to be candidates for more radical surgery, the abdominoperineal resection. Excision of the tumor is performed by using local anesthesia. It is important to inject the anesthetic agent in such a manner that the needle does not penetrate tumor tissue.

In patients with cancers deeply invading the sphincter muscle or involving more than one quadrant of the anal circumference, especially if they are close to the anorectal line, it is necessary to perform abdominoperineal resection. This type of cancer can be eradicated by surgery. However, there are studies in progress, such as the one by Nigro in which a combination of surgery, radiation, and chemotherapy is being used. The results of early cases have been encouraging. Radiation alone has eradicated many early epitheliomas of the anal area. I have several patients who were apparently cured following the therapy outlined by Nigro.

Growths Involving the Anorectal Line. The location of the lesion and its extensions as determined by clinical examination is as important, if not more important, than the histologic appearance. A squamous cell tumor at the anorectal line may present evidence of elements of various cell types occurring in this area of transitional epithelium. The pathologist may occasionally see evidence of mucus-secreting cells, cuboidal in type, instead of the usual appearance of strictly squamous cell carcinoma. Therefore, the term basaloid carcinoma had its origin. Others used different terms, in essence synonyms, such as transitional-cell, cloacogenic, and mucoepidermoid carcinoma, for these lesions. Still others, realizing that these tumors behaved like squamous cell carcinomas, grouped them together as epidermoid cancers or variants of the typical squamous cell cancer.

To put it simply, there are two types of squamous cell cancers at the anorectal area: the true squamous type and those that behave like one. While pathologists may not agree, I treat squamous cell cancer and its variants as one group. It is possible that in the future researchers may break the epidermoid cancer group down into the various histologic variants for determining and comparing survival rates, as Morson has begun to do.

When the anorectal line is involved, the treatment for squamous cell cancer and its variants is abdominoperineal resection. Prophylactic removal of inguinal nodes has no value, and unless the nodes are involved, inguinal node dissection is not performed.

It is important to avoid confusing the easily curable basal cell tumor or rodent ulcer with the potentially lethal basaloid tumor of the anorectal line. Basal cell carcinoma of the anal margin is rare but easily cured by local excision.

Location of the squamous cell tumor of the anorectal area is important in treatment and prognosis. Stearns has reported a 66 per cent five-year survival rate for tumors at or near the anal verge without muscle or nodal involvement. With nodal involvement, according to Goldberg, the five-year survival rate is less than 5 per cent. The overall survival rates are better than expected, being greater than 50 per cent.

ADENOCARCINOMA

Adenocarcinoma of the lower rectum can invade the anal canal, as depicted in Figure 15–5. The tumor may be mistaken, clinically, for squamous cell cancer. The Miles' abdominoperineal resection is indicated.

BOWEN'S DISEASE

According to Strauss and Fazio, this disease presents as a dermatologic problem, which is why the dermatologist sees more of these patients than other specialists. The condition is described as a discrete reddish, plaque-like area with scaly-looking eczematoid features. The appearance of Bowen's disease is so unusual that it should alert the clinician to conduct further investigation. At Memorial Hospital, the treatment of choice is wide, local, full-thickness excision with additional resection of the margins for frozen section to ensure adequate removal. Five out of 12 patients survived 5 to 24 years following surgery. Local excision is reserved for early cases. Invasive lesions require extensive surgical treatment. The advanced case shown in Figure 5-2 would hardly lend itself to any type of surgery, since there were widespread metastases as well as inguinal node involvement.

PERIANAL PAGET'S DISEASE

In reviewing the literature on perianal Paget's disease, Arminski and Pollard state that there were only 32 reported cases up until 1973. Nine patients have been seen at Memorial Hospital. Those lesions with an underlying cancer often present as a mass, and three of the patients seen at Memorial already had inguinal metastases when they were first seen. The lesion is usually distinctive enough to draw attention and invite biopsy. Extramammary Paget's disease may not necessarily be associated with an invasive tumor. At Memorial Hospital, subjacent infiltrating cancer, usually colloid in type, was found in five of nine patients. All these cancers were thought to arise from a perianal gland or other skin appendage and not from the rectal mucosa.

Treatment and prognosis depend on the presence or absence of an underlying invasive carcinoma. According to Stearns, if invasive cancer is not present, local excision is curative. All of the patients at Memorial who had perianal Paget's disease with invasive carcinoma and metastases to the inguinal nodes did poorly and died despite surgical treatment as well as x-ray therapy and chemotherapy. When Paget's disease was associated with early localized invasive cancer, as was seen in one patient, wide local excisions were sufficient to cure the patient. There is one patient who is alive 17 years after the original discovery of the disease even though adenocarcinoma was found 6 and 12 years after the original excision. The recurrence was excised on each occasion.

MELANOMA

If biopsy confirms the diagnosis of melanoma, abdominoperineal resection should be performed as soon as possible. The five-year survival rate is so dismal that every effort should be made to avoid dissemination of the tumor. According to Quan, the isolated reported instances in the medical literature of long-term survivors following local excision of malignant melanoma of the anus indicate that these tumors were very small and unsuspected, and were discovered only after routine examination of tissue removed at hemorrhoidectomy. Quan states that the few good results obtained at Memorial Hospital were due to extensive abdominoperineal resection with pelvic lymph node resection. Only five patients lived beyond the five-year survival mark.

Among the few patients I have seen with malignant melanoma, one patient survived four and one-half years after abdominoperineal resection, at which time the patient developed inguinal node metastases and died shortly afterwards from disseminated disease.

LEIOMYOSARCOMA

Quan reported that in a series of 35 colorectal malignancies at Memorial Hospital the success or failure in the treatment of patients with colorectal leiomyosarcoma is similar to that of carcinoid, in that it is decidedly dependent on the size of the original lesion when first detected. While five patients with rectal leiomyosarcoma of a small size—1 to 2½ cm in diameter at the time of discovery—responded to adequate local excision and are long-term survivals, those with larger tumors—particularly those greater than 6 centimeters—all did poorly regardless of radical surgery and other adjunct treatment modalities.

CARCINOID TUMORS

Only if there is evidence that the tumor is invading the rectal or bowel wall should a carcinoid be considered malignant. Orloff has correlated size of the lesion and evidence of muscle invasion with prognosis. In Orloff's series of 15 carcinoids that were larger than 2 cm in diameter, 13 were invasive, 12 involved the local lymph nodes, and 6 had metastasized to distal organs.

In the clinical management of carcinoids, one must again do a careful examination of the rectum, which begins with a digital examination. The digital examination should not be hurried because practically every small nodule in the rectum or lower portion of the rectum can be palpated with the finger. It is very easy to miss a small carcinoid, just as it is easy to miss any small submucosal nodule or intramucosal nodule. The rectal carcinoids that I have seen showed a yellowish color or at least a yellowish tinge, and I was able to see as well as palpate these little tumors. To put it more vividly, they just look and feel like a small carcinoid in the appendix. In the rectum they are usually 1 cm in diameter, submucosal, and freely movable.

In my experience with biopsy of rectal carcinoids, I find it difficult to perform the procedure in the office without some annoying bleeding, since it is usually necessary to incise the mucosa to reach the involved area. Thus whenever I suspect the presence of a carcinoid in the rectum and provided it is less than 2 cm in diameter, I prefer to give the patient local anesthesia in the hospital and perform an excisional biopsy. In that manner the pathologist will be able to determine whether or not invasion of the muscularis has occurred. However, Quan, who has a vast experience with carcinoids, treated 39 patients with rectal carcinoids on an outpatient basis. I am also sure that some years ago, I fulgurated a few of these nodules without biopsy and without knowing they were carcinoids, just as one would fulgurate tiny mamillations or polyps in the rectum without biopsy. Larger tumors, those over 2 cm, should be considered for resection. A tumor in the rectum over 5 centimeters is generally not a carcinoid; however, there may be exceptions.

Review of the literature indicates that in general the survival rates for patients with colonic carcinoids were poor, but even the largest of the series comprised only 12 patients. I do not believe that 12 patients is a statistically significant experience, even with such a rare condition as carcinoids. Furthermore, these tumors just do not behave as the usual cancer. Various surgeons have noted metastases occurring as long as 13 years after the original operation for a carcinoid tumor in the bowel.

FOLLOW-UP

Cancer of the colon and rectum can be either synchronous or asynchronous. This fact should alert the reader to the importance of thorough initial and follow-up examinations. The patient with colorectal cancer has a good chance of having synchronous cancer, or lesions in other areas of the colon or rectum. Therefore it is important that prior to the initial operation the presence of other cancers or polyps in the colon and rectum is ruled out by x-ray studies and colonoscopy. For some unknown reason, a patient who has had one cancer is prone to develop other cancers either in the same organ or in other organs. His chances of developing cancer at a later time vary from 2 to 9 per cent. Naturally, the longer a patient is followed, the more asynchronous or metachronous cancers will be found. In a highly selected group of patients with cancer of the rectum on whom I performed the pull-through procedure and was able to follow for 20 years, I found that only 4 per cent developed subsequent cancers.

Since recurrence usually occurs during the first two years following surgery, it is advisable to follow the patient very closely during that time. It is important not to wait for symptoms to develop before check-up examinations are performed. In this manner, the patient becomes accustomed to regular examinations and does not live in constant fear of recurrence. A second primary lesion usually does not occur until three or four years after the first resection.

Any signs or symptoms of disease should be noted. Another primary tumor would demonstrate symptoms similar to those manifested by the original lesion. Perineal or pelvic pain is an especially important symptom particularly if it follows abdominoperineal resection. It usually signifies perineural involvement and recurrence of the tumor. Recent studies have shown that electromyography may be of help in detecting early recurrence in the pelvis. The development of a cough could indicate metastases to the lungs or a new primary lesion in the lung. For this reason, a chest x-ray every six months during the first two years is indicated. Persistent headaches could indicate brain metastases. In patients on whom I have performed an anastomosis that is within reach of the sigmoidoscope, I make it a practice to do a sigmoidoscopic examination every three months for the first two years. Lesions requiring anastomoses higher in the colon can be followed with colon x-rays and/or colonoscopic examinations. It is important to conduct baseline study beginning three months after the initial operation, so that if a recurrence develops it can be detected early. Stool examination for occult blood is performed on each visit. These stool tests are much more accurate if performed utilizing an anoscope or sigmoidoscope to obtain the specimen. In this manner, minor conditions at the anorectal area such as hemorrhoids or fissures that could bleed will not confuse the results.

The carcinoembryonic antigen (CEA) test is one method of monitoring patients for recurrent disease. Attiyeh emphasizes that baseline CEA values must be obtained, one prior to surgery and one several months after surgery. Attiyeh advocates performing the CEA test every two to three months in high-risk patients during the first two years. A significant elevation of the CEA should be verified by repeating the test twice in a short period and if the results are consistently high, a further diagnostic work-up is indicated to detect recurrence. A laparotomy may be necessary both to verify and to attempt removal of recurrent disease, although results are dismal.

In practice, it is very difficult to have patients return for even the most routine and practical tests that should be performed. However, there are some patients who demonstrate such anxiety concerning their disease that they request CT and other scans of the liver or other parts of the body. Chest x-rays and blood chemistries need not be ordered more frequently than every six months, although each patient must be considered individually.

REFERENCES

American Joint Committee for Cancer Staging and End-Results Reporting, Manual for Staging of Cancer. J. B. Lippincott Co., Philadelphia, 1983.

Attiyeh, F. F., Personal communication, 1981.

Beart, R., Jr., Personal communication, 1983.

Beart, R. W., Jr., Van Neerden, J. A., and Beahrs, O. H., Evolution in the pathologic staging of carcinoma of the colon. Surg., Gynecol., and Obstet., 146:257–259, 1978.

Bussey, H. J. R., Dukes, C. E., and Lockhar-Mummery, H. E., Results of the surgical treatment of rectal cancer. In Dukes, C. E., ed., Cancer of Cancer of the Rectum. Livingstone, London, 1960.

Corman, M. L., Colon and Rectal Surgery, Philadelphia, J. B. Lippincott Co., 1984.

Goldberg, S. M., Gordon, P. H., and Nivatvongs, S., Essentials of Anorectal Surgery. J. B. Lippincott Co., Philadelphia, 1980.

Grinnell, R. S., The grading and prognosis of carcinoma of the colon and rectum, Annals of Surg., 109:500, 1939.

Grinnell, R. S., Results of ligation of inferior mesenteric artery at the aorta in resection of the descending and sigmoid colon and rectum. Surg., Gynecol., Obstet., 120:1031–1036, 1965.

Jackman, R. J., and Beahrs, O. H., Malignant lymphoma in tumors of the large bowel, W. B. Saunders Co., Philadelphia, 1968, pp. 210–216.

MacKeigan, J. M., and Ferguson, J. A., Prophytactic oophorectomy and colorectal cancer in premenopausal patients. Dis. Colon Rectum 22:401–405, 1979.

Madden, J. L., Personal communication, 1980.

Masson, P., Carcinoids and nerve hyperplasia of appendicular mucosa. Am. J. Pathol., 4:131, 1928.

Mesden, D. D., Shorter, R. G. and Ilsup, D. M., et al., Crohn's disease and cancer. N. Engl. J. Med., 289:1099–1103, 1975.

Nigro, N. D., Vaitkevicius, V. K., and Buroker, T., et al.: Combined therapy for cancer of the anal canal. Dis. Colon Rectum, 24:73–75, 1981.

Novy, S., Rogers, L. F., and Kirkpatrick, W., Diastatic rupture of the cecum in obstructing carcinoma of the left colon: radiographic diagnosis and surgical implications. Am. J. Roentgenol., 121:281–1975.

Orloff, M. J., Carcinoid tumors of the rectum. Cancer, 28:175–180, 1971.

Quan, S. H. Q., and Berg, J. W., Leiomyoma and leiomyosarcoma of the rectum. Dis. Colon Rectum, 5:415, 1962.

Quan, S. H. Q., White, J. E., and Deddish, M. R., Malignant melanoma of the anorectum. Dis. Colon Rectum, 2:275–283, 1959.

Raskin, H., Personal communication, 1973.

Salvati, E. P., and Rubin, R. J., Electrocoagulation as primary therapy for rectal carcinoma. Am. J. Surg., 132:583–586, 1976.

Stearns, M. W., Jr., Neoplasms of the Colon, Rectum and Anus. John Wiley & Sons, New York, 1980.

Strauss, R. J., and Fazio, V. W., Bowen's disease of the anal and perianal area: a report and analysis of 12 cases. Am. J. Surg., 137:231–234, 1979.

Strauss, A. A., Strauss, S. F., Crawford, R. A., and Strauss, H. A., Surgical diathermy of carcinoma of the rectum; its clinical end results. J.A.M.A., 104:1480, 1935.

Turnbull, R. B., Jr., Personal communication, 1976.

Welch, C. E., Personal communication, 1974.

CHAPTER 16

Rare Problems of the Colon and Rectum

INTRODUCTION

The two conditions to be described are rare, constituting only a fraction of problems in the colon or rectum. However, they are formidable and may be life-threatening.

VOLVULUS

Volvulus is a twisting of a redundant loop of intestine on itself to such a degree as to obstruct and frequently compromise the blood supply of the bowel. The redundant bowel twists or rotates around both its base of attachment and the mesenteric pedicle in either a clockwise or a counterclockwise fashion. A rotation of at least 180 degrees must occur before the blood supply is compromised (Figs. 16–1 and 16–2). Although seen anywhere along the gastrointestinal tract, it most frequently occurs in the sigmoid colon. Volvulus accounts for 5 per cent of all cases of intestinal obstruction.

The pathogenesis of volvulus is simple when one considers the predisposing factors involved: a redundant or excessive bowel attached to a relatively narrow base. A redundant sigmoid colon fills the requirements quite well. From a preventative standpoint, a good case can be made for a baseline barium enema examination in all older people. Since constipation for various periods of time precedes acute attacks of volvulus in the sigmoid colon, it might be possible, at least theoretically, for patients with a redundant sigmoid colon to avoid volvulus by avoiding any kind of serious constipation.

Since the obstruction caused by volvulus is acute and complete, the symptoms are rather dramatic. Volvulus is characterized by sudden cramplike abdominal pain, rapid distention of the abdomen, difficulty in breathing because of the pressure on the diaphragm, and, later, nausea and vomiting.

Physical examination of the abdomen shows a tympanitic abdomen. In most cases, the history and radiographic examination will differentiate volvulus from obstruction from any other cause. It is important to order an

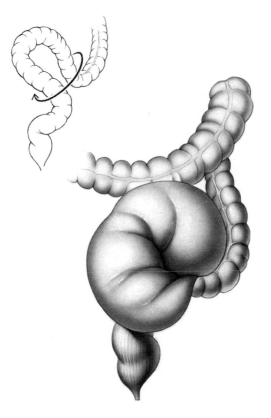

Figure 16–1. Volvulus of the sigmoid colon (360 degrees).

immediate flat plate of the abdomen, which may show a closed, loop-like configuration not unlike a twisted innertube. However, since the proximal large bowel and even the small bowel may be dilated, the diagnosis can be missed. It is therefore important to do a proctosigmoidoscopic examination if a sigmoid volvulus is suspected. If the examination is negative, an emergency RB barium enema examination should be ordered. However, if the proctosigmoidoscopic examination shows obstruction from a suspected twist in the sigmoid colon, nonoperative management should be employed. With the patient in the knee-chest position, a well-lubricated rectal tube should be prepared and an attempt made to pass the rectal tube through the sigmoidoscope into the lumen of the obstructed bowel. This should be done with great caution and with no more pressure than would ordinarily be applied in

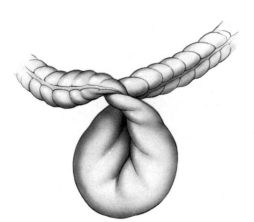

Figure 16–2. Volvulus of the sigmoid colon (180 degrees).

passing a spastic colon or rectosigmoid junction during a usual examination. If passage of the rectal tube is successful and gas as well as liquid stool is obtained, an emergency operation can be prevented, since the rectal tube can be taped in and the bowel prepared with irrigations through the rectal tube. However, before such treatment is followed a flat plate should confirm that the colon has indeed been deflated.

Since volvulus patients are usually elderly and usually have multiple medical problems, they should be prepared as soon as possible for abdominal surgery and primary resection of the sigmoid colon.

If proctosigmoidoscopic examination shows discolored mucosa indicating a compromised blood supply, immediate laparotomy is indicated. The general condition of the patient dictates the extent of the procedure. This might involve merely unwinding the volvulus. However, since most patients with volvulus have rapid recurrence, it is much better to do something more definitive in the way of surgery (Fig. 16–3). Naturally, if the bowel is necrotic, resection is mandatory. If primary anastomosis is not feasible due to dilated bowel and/or poor bowel preparation, then a Hartmann-type of resection, resecting the redundant sigmoid, closing the distal rectum, and bringing out the upper sigmoid or descending colon as a temporary colostomy, would be indicated.

Right colon volvulus presents as an acute small bowel obstruction and demands immediate attention (Fig. 16–4). The patient has acute colicky pain with nausea and vomiting. There is some difference of opinion as to how valuable the barium enema is in the diagnosis. However, in a recent publication Haskin et al. have shown beautiful demonstrations of the diagnosis of right colon volvulus. The flat plate or plain film of the abdomen shows the cecum to be greatly dilated and it may be located anywhere in the abdomen. The distended cecum often assumes a kidney-bean shape. The small bowel shows dilation. The authors suggest that if the plain film findings are equivocal, a low-pressure, slowly administered barium enema is diagnostic. The contrast column may flow to the right colon, demonstrating the spiraling mucosal folds of the twist, or stop in a tapered, beak-like configuration. Depending on the tightness of the twist, some contrast medium may pass

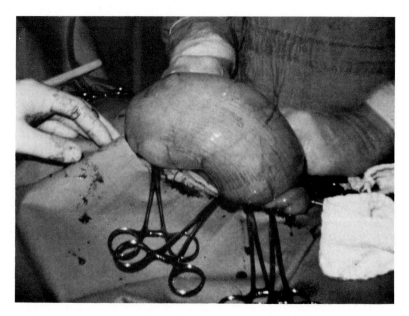

Figure 16–3. Volvulus at surgery (360 degrees).

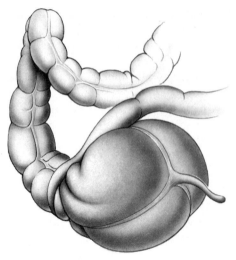

Figure 16–4. Volvulus of cecum.

through the stenotic site into the dilated cecum. In these cases, the spiraling pattern of the volvulated mucosa, best demonstrated on postevacuation film, is pathognomonic.

Early diagnosis is essential, although there is an element of risk in using a barium enema. I have not used the colonoscope for diagnosis; however, potentially such an examination would have the same benefit as the procto-sigmoidoscopic examination in sigmoid volvulus. Of course, enemas would be necessary prior to the examination. Good clinical judgment must be exercised, and in the absence of gangrene, early cases may benefit by such examination.

The treatment is surgical, and when feasible, resection of the redundant ileocecal area is indicated. This should be followed by primary end-to-end anastomosis. Depending on the general medical condition of the patient, one must consider a lesser procedure such as exteriorization over a three-bladed Rankin clamp or simple reduction of the volvulus, attaching the redundant right colon to the lateral peritoneal area. Early diagnosis is stressed because bowel necrosis is associated with an extremely high operative mortality.

PROCIDENTIA OF THE RECTUM

Procidentia, also known as complete prolapse of the rectum, involves all the coats of the rectal wall and is literally a turning inside out of the rectum. (Figs. 16–5 and 16–6). The cul-de-sac extends to the outside beyond the perineum for variable distances; in the female it is not unusual for the uterus and bladder to be involved in the prolapse. The anal sphincter is usually relaxed because of the constant or intermittent stretching caused by prolapse.

Although it is considered a relatively rare disease, it is more commonly seen at the extremes of life. The occurrence of condition in childhood (Fig. 16–7), when the sacrum is a straight bone and before the configuration of concavity has developed, is easily explained. The rectum in early childhood, before the age of 3 years, is a relatively straight tube, and straining exerts pressure directly on the rectum instead of the hollow of the sacrum. Elderly patients, especially those with psychiatric disorders or confined to institutions

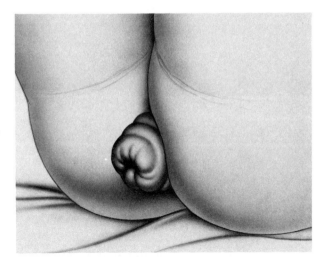

Figure 16–5. Procidentia.

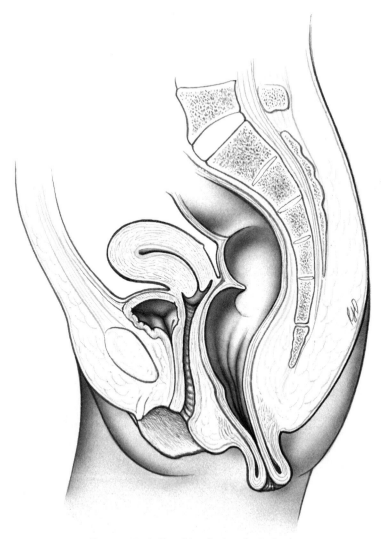

Figure 16–6. Procidentia (sagittal view).

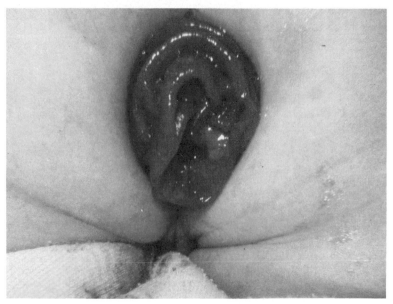

Figure 16–7. Procidentia in a child.

for other reasons, are also prone to the disorder. Muscle weakness and poor bowel habits are contributing factors.

The pathogenesis of procidentia may be either intussusception or sheer perineal muscle weakness. The pathogenesis does not change the treatment of the disease. There is a rather rare condition that may be confused with procidentia in which the sigmoid colon only is intussuscepted into the rectum and may extend out through the anal sphincters (Fig. 16–8). The condition does not involve the rectal wall and is easily recognized. In my experience, the cause of this rare type of intussusception is a tumor in the sigmoid colon, and sigmoidectomy is indicated.

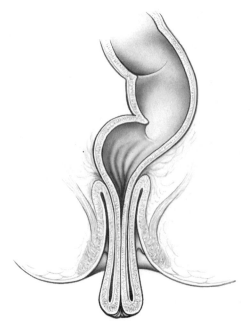

Figure 16–8. Intussusception of sigmoid colon beyond the anus.

TREATMENT

For years, surgeons did not have a successful treatment for procidentia. Many operations were proposed, none of which were satisfactory except the anterior resection and the sling operation of Ripstein in patients who could tolerate an abdominal operation. A variety of surgical procedures still exists. In a 1981 survey of Fellows of the American Society of Colon and Rectal Surgeons, 63.5 per cent favored the Ripstein procedure and 23.5 per cent selected a procedure involving resection as their choice of surgery for procidentia. Others listed operations performed by the perineal approach and not involving abdominal surgery. A few responses indicate that surgeons were trying to simplifly the Ripstein procedure to avoid mobilization of the rectum.

Similarly, many perineal procedures were described for elderly and poor-risk patients. It remained for Altemeier in 1952 to describe a safe and effective operation for this type of patient. Some surgeons have reported a recurrence rate of 23 per cent following the Altemeier procedure, although Altemeier and others who have performed this operation have claimed recurrence rates of 5 per cent or less.

ANTERIOR RESECTION

The technic of anterior resection is basically the same as that described for cancer of the upper rectum (p. 208). For procidentia this approaches the ideal treatment, removing the redundant sigmoid and upper rectum that is created after mobilization of the rectum. All the "slack" is literally eliminated from the sigmoid colon and rectum. It is not necessary to make any attempts at stabilizing the rectum by sutures. Such attempts are not only unnecessary but invite iatrogenic conditions such as bleeding or fistula formation. The anastomosis in anterior resection for procidentia is seldom low, since when the prolapsed rectum is properly mobilized and "straightened out," the anastomosis can usually be made at the level of the sacral promontory.

I have used the anterior resection for many years, and I know of no recurrences of procidentia following the operation. Anterior resection avoids the potential complication of volvulus due to redundant sigmoid. I also prefer to avoid mesh or any foreign substance in any operation unless there is no substitute.

RIPSTEIN PROCEDURE

This is the most simple and most popular abdominal operation for procidentia. The operation consists of mobilization of rectum and fixation of the rectum to the hollow of the sacrum utilizing a strip of Teflon or Marlex mesh. A collar 5 cm wide is made from the mesh in such a manner that it acts as a sling surrounding the anterior and lateral portions of the mobilized rectum. Each end is sutured to the presacral fascia and periosteum of the sacrum approximately 5 cm below the promontory of the sacrum. Data on the results of 1111 Ripstein procedures have been obtained by Gordon and Hoexter (Table 16–1).

Treatment for Poor-Risk Patients

THE THIERSCH OPERATION

The Thiersch operation, in which a wire or plastic strand is placed around the anal canal to retain the procidentia, is seldom satisfactory. The wire

Table 16–1. RESULTS OF 1111 RIPSTEIN PROCEDURES*

Condition	No. of Patients	% Recurrence
Recurrences	26	2.3
Complications	183	16.6
Fecal impaction	74	6.7
Presacral hemorrhage	29	2.6
Stricture	20	1.8
Pelvic abscess	17	1.5
Small bowel obstruction	15	1.4
Impotence	9	0.8
Fistula	4	0.4
Miscellaneous	15	1.4

*From Goldberg, S., Gordon, P. H., and Nivatvongs, S., Essentials of Anorectal Surgery. J. B. Lippincott Co., Philadelphia, 1980.

usually breaks or erodes through the skin after a variable period of time. Fecal impactions may also be related directly to this procedure. Its simplicity recommends it for poor-risk patients, but it seldom relieves the condition over a period of months or years.

This procedure can be done in the office or hospital. After preparation of the immediate perianal area, a local anesthetic is injected and a small skin incision is made approximately one inch posteriorly as well as anteriorly to the anal musculature. A strand of No. 28 silver wire is used. Although the smaller caliber wire ties with a less prominent knot, with less potential for eroding through the skin, it breaks more easily. The wire may easily be introduced with a large needle such as is used for through-and-through abdominal closures. The needle is inserted deeply in the subcutaneous tissues through one incision and out through the second incision. The needle is reinserted through the same incision to circle the other half of the anal canal and out through the original incision. The suture is tied so that the anus admits only the tip of the index finger. The incisions are closed with one or two fine Prolene sutures. No special preparation is needed for this operation. It is important to have the anus tight enough to avoid any prolapse, with possible strangulation. The disadvantages of the Thiersch operation are recurrence when the wire breaks and fecal impaction.

THE ALTEMEIER PROCEDURE

Most elderly and poor-risk patients can tolerate a definitive operation for procidentia by the perineal approach. The Altemeier procedure, performed under some type of regional anesthesia or even with local anesthesia, is a safe and effective operation. The preparation is similar to that used for any resection, although it can be performed following simple preparation utilizing only enemas. The jack-knife position used for the majority of anorectal procedures is satisfactory and even has advantages in that it facilitates surgery and when the cul-de-sac is opened, the small bowel tends to "fall away" from the operative field.

The operation is usually performed with the patient under spinal anesthesia. A Foley catheter is usually used during the procedure and left in the bladder for three to five days postoperatively. With the patient in the jack-knife position, the area is prepared with Betadine. The prolapsed rectal mass is brought to its maximum protrusion with the aid of Babcock forceps. An incision is then made in the rectal wall of the outer layer about 3 to 4 cm proximal to the anorectal line. The incision is performed throughout the entire circumference, and the bleeding points tied with triple 0 chromic catgut suture. The first layer of the bowel is then stripped distally from the underlying or inner loop. The hernial sac is then located anteriorly and dissected free superiorly in its entire circumference as far as possible. The sac is opened and the peritoneal cavity explored. The sliding character of the hernia becomes apparent, because the posterior peritoneal layer of the sac is the serosa of the rectum. A large redundant loop of rectum and the sigmoid colon with attached messentery is visualized and easily delivered into the wound. The site of resection of excess bowel is then selected so that the anastomosis can be made later without tension or redundancy. The mesocolon and its vessels are divided at the selected site, and the bowel prepared for resection and anastomosis. The peritoneal cavity is closed by suturing the peritoneum anteriorly. The obliteration of the cul-de-sac is accomplished at a high level in this manner.

The bowel is then retracted posteriorly and the levator ani muscles are exposed on both sides. Their edges are then approximated anteriorly in the midline with three to four interrupted sutures of 0 chromic catgut. The redundant bowel is then divided into two halves by cutting it anteriorly and posteriorly up to the point of anastomosis. This is important in order to prevent retraction of the bowel into the pelvis. The anastomosis is begun by placing 0 chromic sutures through the full thickness of rectal cuff and sigmoid colon. This is allowed to remain long as a guy suture. A similar suture is placed anteriorly and this is also allowed to remain long. One half of the redundant bowel is then transected progressively. The anastomosis completed with interrupted sutures of the same material until the entire circumference of the bowel and anal mucosa or rectal cuff has been united. The anastomotic area retracts easily into the rectum. The patients are ambulatory and eating a regular diet by the next day.

These patients do extremely well regardless of their age, and I have had some as old as 97 years. However, many patients have a tendency to diarrhea and poor control, and it is important to be understanding and tolerant of this because their adjustment is extremely slow. The only other problem encountered in this age group is bladder dysfunction. However, both problems seem to resolve with time, except in a few extremely senile patients.

REFERENCES

Altemeier, W. A., Ginseffi, J., and Hoxworth, P., Treatment of extensive prolapse of the rectum in aged or debilitated patients. Arch. Surg., 65:72–80, 1952.

Gordon, P. H., and Hoexter, B., Complications of the Ripstein procedure. Dis. Colon Rectum, 21:277–280, 1978.

Haskin, P. H., Teplick, S. K., Teplick, J. G., and Haskin, M. E., Volvulus of the cecum and right colon. J.A.M.A., 245:2433–2435, 1981.

Ripstein, C. B., Procidentia: definitive corrective surgery. Dis. Colon Rectum, 15:334–336, 1972.

CONSTIPATION

INTRODUCTION

Constipation is an affliction of civilization. It is unknown to the animal living in its natural environment; proper food and the exercise expended in foraging for it unwittingly supply adequate stimuli for natural intestinal motility. The colon responds to bulk by increased motility, and the formed stool that is evacuated on a daily basis provides the sphincter muscles of the anal canal with exercise by the process of gentle dilation.

For many years, scientists have known and studied the action of bulk on the colon and anal canal. It is only recently that this knowledge has begun to be appreciated and applied properly in the prevention and treatment of functional and organic colorectal diseases. It is possible that increasing the amount of dietary fiber to prevent and manage constipation may also aid in the prevention of diseases such as diverticulitis and colorectal cancer. There are some who would take exception to this simplistic approach to colorectal disease. They may not believe that bulk is an adequate stimulus for the colon and that the passage of a formed stool provides the only satisfactory exercise required by the sphincter muscles. However, the fact cannot be ignored that both constipation and anorectal disease are unknown in lower animals, in which adequate stools are the rule rather than the exception.

CLASSIFICATION

The question of whether constipation is a symptom or a disease is not altogether clear. It may be best to think of constipation as a symptom in some instances and a disease in others. Constipation may be a primary disease of the colon or occur secondary to anorectal or systemic disease. It may be functional or organic in origin. For these reasons, constipation does not lend itself to a simple approach in classification. The following common varieties will be discussed separately, with the knowledge that some degree of overlap and confusion will occur until a more logical classification evolves:

1. Simple or primary constipation.
2. Constipation secondary to anorectal disease.
3. Constipation secondary to systemic disease.
4. Constipation due to medication.
5. Constipation due to immobilization.
6. Psychogenic constipation.

DIAGNOSIS AND MANAGEMENT

Simple or Primary Constipation

Simple or primary constipation is the most frequent type encountered. History and physical examination with the proctosigmoidoscope quickly make the diagnosis. The patients are frequently young and otherwise healthy individuals. Older patients will require complete investigation of the colon by means of barium enema or colonoscopic examination. The history will usually reveal irregular eating and bowel habits, with failure to eat breakfast and a lack of bulk in the diet.

All examinations are usually negative. Proper diet and a regular habit of elimination after breakfast each morning are essential. Sometimes one or more glycerin suppositories must be inserted in the rectum to prompt a bowel movement at the proper time. Occasionally a small instillation of water by means of a rubber ear syringe is necessary to initiate evacuation. The ear syringe is harmless in that there are no detachable parts that can be lost in the rectum. Good habits can be established in this manner, and within a few months, defecation occurs each morning without the aid of a suppository or enema.

Constipation Secondary to Anorectal Disease

Physiology of Defecation. Normally the entire gastrointestinal tract is like an assembly line, where contents of various consistency occupy the entire length of the tract. Selective digestion and absorption is a constant process throughout the length of the gastrointestinal tract.

Food in the stomach is relatively solid and gradually becomes more liquid as it proceeds into the small intestine. Food material is broken down into suitable units for absorption within the small intestine. The remaining liquid and fiber enters the colon, where water and certain salts are absorbed. In other words, we "eat" with the small bowel and "drink" with the large bowel. The intestinal contents become increasingly solid or bulky as they proceed distally in the colon.

Although any of these processes may change with circumstances, just before defecation the solid contents of the sigmoid colon are rapidly passed into the rectum by action of the gastrocolic reflex. Defecation occurs because of strong peristaltic action and relaxation of the sphincter mechanism, with augmentation by voluntary straining. After defecation, the rectum should be empty.

Unfortunately, some people, because of perineal muscular weakness such as is caused by a rectocele, anal strictures, or anal fissures, find it difficult or are unable to expel the stool. This condition is known as *dyschezia*. It may be so severe that the dry, bulky stool accumulates in the rectum. The patient may succeed in only frequent partial evacuations or evacuate only mucus and blood from straining. The latter condition is known as frequency from overflow, as occurs occasionally in an overdistended bladder.

In spite of perineal weakness, the patient may compensate for this deficiency by being especially careful to have a regular stool at the optimum time, which is after breakfast. Temporarily, it may even be necessary to insert a glycerin suppository in the rectum or use a small instillation of tap water to prompt the stool. Such measures may be necessary until the underlying anatomic deficiency causing the stagnation of stool can be corrected. Definitive management includes repair of the rectocele or correction of painful conditions such as a fissure or anal contraction.

Organic Disease. A frequent cause of constipation is organic disease. Anorectal disease such as fissures and strictures or varying degrees of contraction make it difficult for the patient to evacuate a normal stool due to either pain or the mechanical problem of a contracted anal canal.

It is important that one does not jump to the conclusion that anorectal disease is the only problem. Fissures and other anorectal disease are very common and may occur simultaneously with a tumor or other organic disease higher in the rectum or colon. A good rule to follow is to perform a proctosigmoidoscopic examination on all patients. A small-caliber pediatric scope, well lubricated with 5 per cent lidocaine (Xylocaine) ointment can be introduced into the anal canal in 95 per cent of patients with fissures and strictures. This scope is 12 inches long and makes it possible to examine the entire lower sigmoid. In older patients or those with symptoms suggesting disease higher in the colon, the entire colon should be examined by barium enema or colonoscopy using the narrow-caliber colonoscope.

When the diagnosis is finally made and found to be that of chronic anal fissure with or without anal contraction as the cause of the constipation, the matter should be discussed with the patient. Surgery is indicated. Such patients usually have considerable pain. If large hemorrhoids are present, hemorrhoidectomy should be performed at the same time.

A scar causing anal contraction may follow radical hemorrhoidectomy. In severe cases the anal outlet may be so contracted that it may hardly admit the tip of a lead pencil. However, this scar seldom involves more than the skin of the anal verge and my easily be relieved by utilizing local anesthesia and incising the scar in one or more quadrants of the anal canal (Fig. 17–1A). After release of this "piano wire"-like scar surrounding the lower portion of the anal canal (Fig. 17–1B), the patient's relief is dramatic. The sphincter can expand to an almost-normal diameter, and normal bowel movements follow. However, it is good policy to follow these patients in the office at weekly intervals. During these visits, the index finger should be inserted in the anal canal until normal formed stools accomplish natural dilation. Increasing the amount of bulk in the diet is important. In these and similar cases, the contraction must be relieved before the proctosigmoidoscope can be introduced for more detailed inspection. All of these patients, except those with unusually severe hemorrhoidal disease or severe systemic disease, may be managed in an outpatient setting.

Strictures that cause constipation occur higher in the rectum and colon, and are relatively frequent. Cancers causing various degrees of obstruction are more prevalent in the left colon or rectosigmoid, where the diameter of the bowel is appreciably less than on the right side. It is for this reason that patients 35 years of age and older and all patients with symptoms suggesting this possibility should have a complete investigation of the lower bowel, consisting of a yearly sigmoidoscopic examination and a barium enema or colonoscopic examination at least every three years. Biopsy confirms the diagnosis.

Patients with malignancy may present with gradual onset of abdominal distress and constipation. Occasionally, a patient may note the onset of sudden obstruction and cannot pass flatus or stool. The flat plate shows

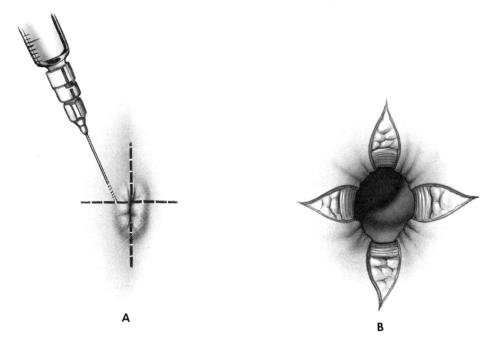

A

B

Figure 17–1. Treatment of contracted anal opening. *A,* Injection of local anesthetic agent. *B,* The annular scar has been incised in all 4 quadrants.

distention of the colon with air and stool. If enemas fail to relieve this problem and proctosigmoidoscopy reveals a cancer, it is sometimes possible to pass a rectal tube through the narrowed area and tape it to the buttocks. This must be done under direct vision and using a Buie biopsy forceps to gently maneuver the well-lubricated tip of the rectul tube through the strictured area (Fig. 17–2). The tube will pass easily, if at all, and force must not be used. If the maneuver is successful, the patient will have been saved a temporary colostomy and may be prepared for an elective resection.

Benign strictures of the rectum or colon that cause constipation are not common but they do occur. Biopsy may cause annoying bleeding and should not be performed unless there is a strong suspicion of malignant degeneration in long-standing cases or evidence of invasion of the rectum by extrarectal cancer. Benign strictures require the use of mineral oil by mouth to keep the stools liquid to avoid fecal impaction and obstruction.

Radiation strictures occur in the rectum at times, following radiation therapy for cervical lesions. The associated radiation proctitis is easily recognized. Malignant or suspected malignant degeneration of a radiation stricture of the rectum requires extirpation of the rectum. Figure 17–3 shows a surgical specimen of a malignant stricture in a rectum severely injured by radiation. Strictures secondary to ulcerative colitis, Crohn's disease, and lymphogranuloma venereum are discussed with those conditions in other sections of this book.

Hirschsprung's Disease. Hirshsprung's disease is a congenital disease characterized by absence of ganglion cells in the rectum, therefore causing atony and contraction of the rectosigmoid with dilatation of the proximal colon. Symptoms occur early in neonatal life. Congenital megacolon is an appropriate synonym for this condition because of the enormous dilatation of the colon. The abdomen is extremely protuberant. Hirschsprung's disease is a chronic condition. A colostomy should be performed as a preliminary

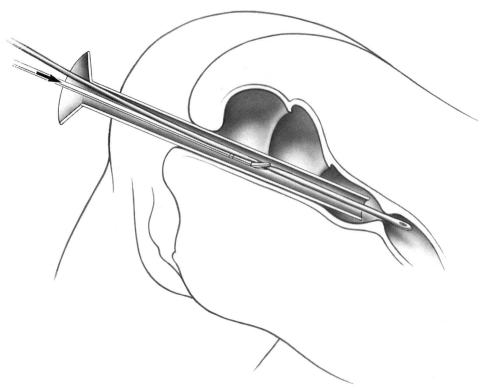

Figure 17–2. Inserting a rectal tube through an obstructing lesion of the colon.

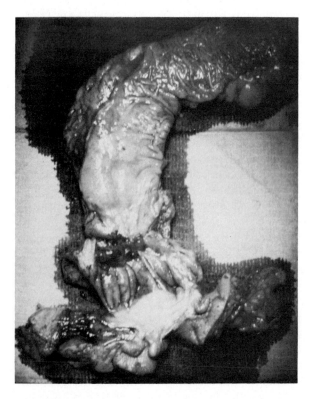

Figure 17–3. Specimen of malignant stricture in rectum resulting from radiation proctitis.

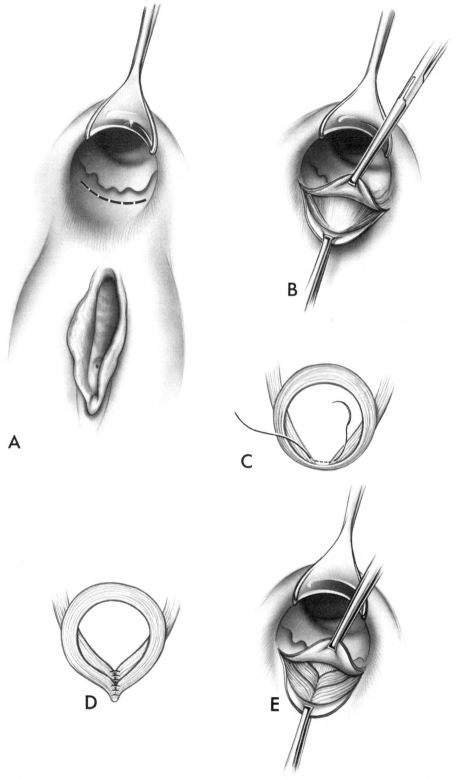

Figure 17–4. Repair of a weak perineum. *A,* Transverse incision below the dentate line. *B,* Raising skin and mucosal flap reveals the thin perineum as well as the normal levator and sphincter muscles. *C,* Repair of levator muscle by interrupted sutures. *D,* Repair of sphincter muscle by interrupted sutures. *E,* Complete repair of muscles. Skin flaps will be reunited by sutures.

measure, followed by definitive resection of the rectum with anastomosis after the child gains weight and otherwise improves. These problems are best managed by the pediatric surgeon.

Rectocele. Generally speaking, a rectocele is repaired by the gynecologist using a surgical approach to the rectovaginal septum from the vaginal side. However, the proctologic surgeon is frequently faced with the problem of a "thin" perineum and rectocele following a childbirth injury. The deficiency is a partially destroyed anal sphincter anteriorly, with separation of the levator muscles, which allows the rectum to bulge into the vagina.

Such a condition can be corrected quite simply by a transverse incision, one or two inches in length, just distal to the anorectal line (Fig. 17–4A). The skin flap is raised and the sphincter and levator muscles exposed anteriorly and on either side to permit repair (Fig. 17–4B). The levators are brought together anteriorly by a series of interrupted catgut or fine wire sutures until a strong perineal body has been constructed (Fig. 17–4C). The sphincter muscle is then reinformed by a similar process (Fig. 17–4D), and the skin is closed and the operation completed (Fig. 17–4E).

Fecal Impaction. A firm rock-like piece of stool in the rectum may mimic a tumor or even diarrhea because of rectal tenesmus. Careful examination is necessary to determine the extent of the impaction. Abdominal examination may reveal firm stool in various portions of the colon. Occasionally, even the small bowel or at least the distal portion of the colon may be involved (Fig. 17–5).

Administering castor oil by mouth is dangerous because of the possibility of causing a perforation of the colon in areas of ulceration caused by the impacted stool. It is frequently possible to break up the hard stool with the finger. Care is necessary to avoid trauma to the rectum by this procedure. Lacerations and even abscesses may be caused by traumatic removal of impactions. There is no great hurry in breaking up the impaction. Mineral oil enemas several times a day for several days will eventually soften the inspissated stool, providing the oil is retained (Fig. 17–6). Frequently, the anus has lost its tone to varying degrees simply from fatigue due to pressure from impacted stool, and retention of fluid of any kind is difficult. In such cases and others, using the knee-chest position or left lateral Sims' position can be of great help. Persistence is the key to successful resolution of fecal impaction.

Constipation Due to Systemic Disease

Diabetes, lead poisoning, and uremia are frequent causes of constipation. Treatment of the underlying disease is indicated.

Constipation Due to Medication

There are many medications that affect peristalsis and cause constipation. Sedatives, opiates, and anticholinergics are some of the more common ones. Discontinuation of such medication usually relieves the constipation.

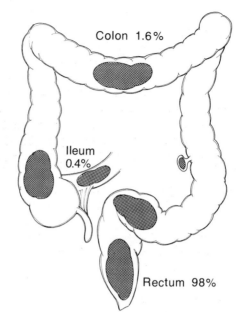

Figure 17–5. Sites of fecal impaction.

Colon 1.6%

Ileum
0.4%

Rectum 98%

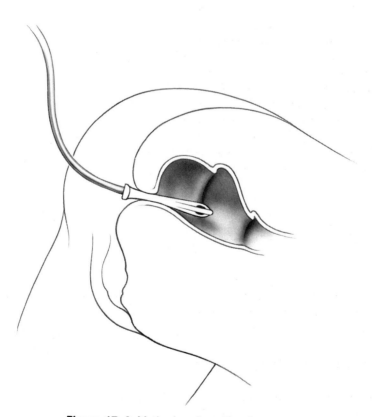

Figure 17–6. Method and position for enema.

Constipation Due to Immobilization

Bed rest due to cardiac disease, fractures, and other afflictions requiring prolonged immobilization is a frequent cause of constipation and makes strict attention to bowel function a necessity.

Psychogenic Constipation

Inanition and associated medications are a frequent cause of constipation in psychotic patients. These patients are likely to have anorexia and are particularly apt to develop impactions. Frequent digital examinations are necessary to diagnose impending impactions. Depending on the circumstances, either enemas or laxatives are necessary.

CHAPTER 18

DIET

INTRODUCTION

There are many who attribute good health solely to one's genes, and there is some truth to this. However, in performing colonoscopy on many patients of various ages and for various reasons, one gains the distinct impression that there must be a way to modify or even prevent the development of such diseases as diverticular disease.

The colon normally is a mobile organ consisting of smooth muscle. The colon needs exercise as do the other muscles. The adequate stimulus for movement is bulk. Many of the patients referred to me provide a history of lack of bulk-producing foods in the diet. They will frequently state that they do not like fibrous or whole-grain foods; they may even claim that such foods do not "agree" with them. In other words, they have been using highly refined foods for many years and their colons are unaccustomed to handling bulk. The principle involved is atrophy from disuse. Even if they do not develop diverticular disease, such patients are apt to have spastic colons with frequent stools. Adequate bulk would tend to keep the colon moderately distended and thus prevent the terrific spasms accounting for their abdominal pains and diarrhea.

Bulk alone is not the complete answer to these patients' problems, since the addition of artificial bulk does not always correct their condition. The nutrition in natural bulk foods does seem to be essential, however, not only for health of the colon but for general health. By the same reasoning, a high-fiber diet may have a preventive effect on the pathogenesis of cancer, colitis, and other colorectal diseases, as well as general disease.

DIET AND ANORECTAL DISEASE

For the most part, dietary principles have been discussed in association with specific diseases such as fissure and hemorrhoids. As described previously, the rectal outlet is composed of both involuntary and voluntary muscle. The levator and external sphincter muscles are composed of voluntary muscle and the internal sphincter muscle consists of involuntary muscle. Both need the exercise provided by a formed stool passing through the outlet each day. This will prevent atrophy, in which the normal muscle is replaced by fibrous tissue that causes bands of contraction.

Most acute fissures will respond to a high-bulk diet, which in turn results in formed stools. Acute fissures should heal in four to five weeks. Recently, it has been found that the "healing" trace metal zinc in a dose of 50 mg daily after a meal is of great help. A few patients cannot tolerate this medication and should avoid it if this is the case. It is seldom necessary to take laxatives for the cure of fissures, and adequate amounts of bulk-producing foods are much more desirable. Most subacute and chronic fissures that are associated with variable degrees of anal contraction require surgery for cure. Temporary use of mineral oil by mouth, milk of magnesia, or a combination of both may be necessary to help relieve the pain until definitive treatment can be planned.

Hemorrhoids, which consist of clumps of veins containing stagnant blood, may be caused or at least aggravated by a tight sphincter muscle, which can conceivably be caused by lack of formed stools. The adequate stimulus for maintaining a lumen of normal caliber for the rectal outlet is the regular passage of a formed stool. Lord of England was perhaps the first to make this observation, and he advocated anal dilatation under general anesthesia as the treatment of choice of hemorrhoids. Although his treatment has not become popular, the principle behind it is good. Anatomically, it is better practice to sever the band causing the contraction under local anesthesia (see p. 96).

The attempt to relieve hemorrhoids by something short of a complete hemorrhoidectomy signifies a healthy trend of treating anorectal problems in a more conservative fashion. Prevention in the form of proper diet, exercise, proper bowel habits, and the practice of good anal hygiene is taking the lead in the management of hemorrhoids and many other anorectal problems.

DIET AND COLON DISEASE

Diets high in residue and low in cholesterol are generally considered part of a preventative regime for such diseases as colon cancer, colitis, and diverticulitis. However, when cancer has developed to such a point where a "napkin-ring" lesion has caused constriction or narrowing of the lumen, a high-residue or -bulk diet may actually precipitate an obstruction. In such cases, it is best to avoid bulk and even have the patient take mineral oil by mouth to keep the stools liquid or soft until definitive surgery can be planned. By following such a course it may be possible to prevent a staged procedure, that is, a colostomy followed by resection.

Another circumstance in which modified diet or nutritional support would be indicated on a temporary basis is an exacerbation of colitis. In such cases a clear-liquid diet or even parenteral nutrition or hyperalimentation might be indicated to put the bowel at complete rest.

Acute diverticulitis poses a similar problem. In the presence of an acutely inflamed bowel, it is best to avoid any nourishment by mouth on a temporary basis, that is, until the fever and symptoms are controlled. The terms "putting the bowel at rest" or "splinting" the bowel are synonymous. This will afford an opportunity to observe the patient closely for progress or the lack of it. Furthermore, if emergency surgery should prove necessary, the bowel will be relatively clean, which in itself would make surgical complications less likely to occur.

REFERENCE

Lord, P. H., Conservative management of hemorrhoids. Part II: Dilatation treatment. Clin. Gastroenterol., 4:601, 1975.

Index

Note: Page numbers in *italic* type indicate illustrations; page numbers followed by *t* refer to tables.